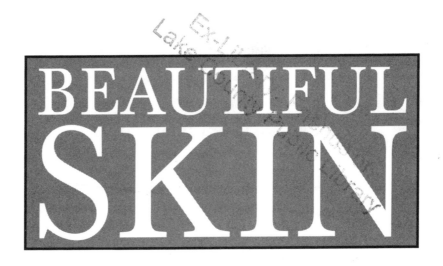

BEAUTIFUL SKIN

EVERY WOMAN'S GUIDE TO LOOKING HER BEST AT ANY AGE

David E. Bank, M.D.

with Estelle Sobel

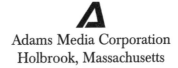

Adams Media Corporation
Holbrook, Massachusetts

3 3113 01883 2859

Published by
Adams Media Corporation
260 Center Street, Holbrook, MA 02343. U.S.A.

ISBN: 1-58062-325-5

Printed in the United States of America.

J I H G F E D C B A

Library of Congress Cataloging-in-Publication Data
Bank, David, M.D.
Beautiful skin / by David Bank, with Estelle Sobel.
p.   cm.
ISB 1-58062-325-5
1. Skin–Care and hygiene. I. Sobel, Estelle. II. Title.
RL87.B34 2000
646.7'26–dc21   00-02629

The illustrations on pages 5, 6, and 7 are reprinted by permission from the National Rosacea Society, Barrington, IL.

The illustrations on pages 38 and 39 by Roberta Collier-Morales.

The illustration on page 68 is reprinted by permission of The Skin Cancer Foundation, from the brochure *The ABCD's of Moles & Melanomas*, copyright 1985, The Skin Cancer Foundation, New York, NY.

Photo on page 98 courtesy of ©Stockbyte Royalty Free Photos.

Many of the designations used by manufacturers and sellers to distinguish their products are claimed as trademarks. Where those designations appear in this book and Adams Media was aware of a trademark claim, the designations have been printed in initial capital letter (e.g., Neutrogena).

This publication is designed to provide accurate and authoritative information with regard to the subject matter covered. It is sold with the understanding that the publisher is not engaged in rendering professional medical advice. If assistance is required, the services of a competent professional person should be sought.

This book is available at quantity discounts for bulk purchases.
For information, call 1-800-872-5627.

Visit our exciting Web site: www.adamsmedia.com

Table of Contents

Acknowledgments

Dr. David E. Bank's Acknowledgments

I gratefully acknowledge my co-author Estelle Sobel, whose hard work, late hours, and great ideas were invaluable to this book. Likewise, Katharine Sands, my literary agent, who so aptly guided me through the process of bringing this book to fruition. I am indebted to my staff and colleagues at The Center for Dermatology, Cosmetic and Laser Surgery for their input and opinions: Dr. Cynthia Gerardi, Dr. Maritza Perez, Dr. Grace Pak, Dr. Douglass Monasebian, Dolores Croce, Brian DeToma, Jill Fazzinga, Lisa Feeney, Janice Iodice, Kathryn Larson, Kathleen Raneri, Ellen Starace, and especially Pam Ferraro. I thank the professionals whose contributions appear in this book as well as many other friends and colleagues that gave me their opinions and support.

Thanks must also go to Bob Adams and the fabulous team at Adams Media, especially Paula Munier-Lee, Linda Spencer, Dawn Thompson, and Carrie Lewis for all their help in making this dream become a reality.

I especially want to give my thanks and my love to my wonderful family: My wife Randee and my two sons, Michael and Alex.

Estelle Sobel's Acknowledgments

I am grateful for the professional expertise, hard work, and friendship of my co-author Dr. David E. Bank. I'd also like to thank my literary agent, Katharine Sands, of Sarah Jane Freymann Literary Agency for her savvy guidance and boundless enthusiasm for this book. I am indebted to my support team: My parents, Miriam and Jerry Sobel, my sister, Michelle Margolis, Kenny Fakler, Irina Harris, and my Colorado connections: Phyllis Sutherland, Beth Bennett, and especially Tom Bennett. A big thank-you must also go to Pam Ferraro for her invaluable assistance and to all the professionals who contributed to this book. A special thanks to Paula Munier-Lee, our wonderful editor, and also grateful thanks to the following people at Adams Media: Carrie Lewis, Dawn Thompson, Linda Spencer, Susan Beale, Chris Ciaschini, Paul Beatrice, Colleen Sell.

Introduction

Life shrinks or expands in proportion to one's courage.

–Anaïs Nin

Dear Reader:

You've bought this book for a reason. We know what that reason is–you want to look better, a lot better, right now. And why shouldn't you? In today's society, a good first impression is crucial. Many women and men, regardless of their age, occupation, or social class, are judged not only by how they act, but also by how they look.

That's why *Beautiful Skin* offers a program to beautify every skin type and to help you find the simplest, least expensive answer to any skin care or cosmetic problem, whether you are Black, Asian, Latino, or Caucasian.

Today, the public is flooded with such a barrage of information–much of it inaccurate and misleading–that people often feel overwhelmed. Sifting through it all to separate what is real from what is hype can be mind-boggling. My job is to simplify the complicated and to offer you a scientific plan for looking, and ultimately feeling, better that is based on proven, cutting-edge techniques and is specifically suited to your age, skin type, nationality, and diet.

Throughout the book I cover all the questions I receive daily from beauty editors of publications such as *The New York Times, Elle, Mirabella, Family Circle, Health, Self, Redbook, Bazaar, Cosmopolitan, Glamour, Fitness, McCall's, W, Allure,* and *Teen People,* who rely on me for the most comprehensive and timely information available. I'll do for you what I do for them: boil down the information into a sound, medically correct solution or procedure.

I want you to know everything I know about how to make your skin look, feel, and stay its best. In every chapter, you'll find tons of fast facts, Web sites, research data, and advice that will help you determine the best beauty and health options available to you. You'll find between these covers a complete program for improving your appearance and the health of your skin in every way: from fixing dark under-eye circles to reducing wrinkles, and finding the right products to smooth, tighten, and heal your skin. This comprehensive beauty and skin care program, along with the accompanying helpful tips, encompasses every type of skin and skin texture, whether young or old, smooth or wrinkled, normal, oily, dry, or combination, acne-prone, ruddy, or sensitive. You even get a head-to-toe guide to the latest and tried-and-true products, potions, and treatments available—from Retin-A to glycolic acid. This product and procedure guide also provides advice on which treatments work and which don't, the latest in laser therapy, the kinds of wrinkles that respond better to Botox than to collagen or peels, which procedures should be done by a dermatologist rather than a plastic surgeon (you'll be surprised), and the real scoop on a host of other skin-related procedures questioned by women everywhere.

There's no doubt about it: feeling good about the way you look gives you an edge when it comes to getting ahead in life. Many therapists tell their patients to "act as if they are happy" and eventually they will feel a sense of happiness. That's very basic, but the same premise applies to your appearance. When you feel good about yourself, you can't help but transmit that happiness to everyone you meet, whether in your professional, social, or home life.

Beautiful Skin is your one-stop shopping guide and program for a more beautiful, younger-looking, and healthier you. We are in an information age— and information is power. Look at this book as your very own manual for navigating, understanding, and applying the latest information and advancements in skin health and beauty. If I've done my job correctly, I will have helped you to look and feel your best, by providing you with everything you need to know to make the soundest skin-care decisions—without your having to spend hundreds of hours searching and downloading from the Web, clipping magazines, or scouring through medical journals—in a very personal house call from me.

As I always say, "It's not what you spend, it's knowing what you're buying."

Let's begin.

chapter one

Beauty House Call

He has half the deed done, who has made a beginning.
—HORACE

DO YOU WONDER WHAT SHAPE YOUR SKIN IS IN? WHEN YOU LOOK IN THE MIRROR, does it appear smooth and blemish-free? Or is it blotchy and blemished? Does your skin look healthy?–or does your skin seem pasty and lacking in tone?

What about your skin-care routine? Is it meeting your needs? Or do you wake up in the morning and see oily stains on your pillow, either from skin that's too oily or from a moisturizer that's not doing its job properly? Do you find that when winter comes your skin gets dry and scratchy, and your regular moisturizer doesn't seem to work anymore?

Whatever your answers, take comfort in the fact that you're not alone. First of all, you may want to take this simple tissue test to determine whether your skin fits into one of the four major categories: oily, combination, normal, or dry. Keep in mind that as the seasons change, the texture and condition of your skin will change with them too.

The Tissue Test

- Wash your face, but don't use moisturizer afterward.
- Wait 15 minutes and then use a tissue to blot your entire face.
- Now look at the tissue:

If you see oily spots all over the tissue, you have oily skin. Other signs of oily skin are visible pores and an orange-peel-like texture.

If the T-zone (forehead and nose) of your skin transfers oil onto the tissue, you have combination skin, which also shows up as a cross between dehydrated cheeks and an oily T-zone.

If you have little to no oil diffusely all over, you have normal skin. It is uniform and homogeneous throughout the face (not a split like combination skin with an oily T-zone and dry cheeks). It does not overly react to products or external factors and does not break out excessively.

If the tissue turns up blotch-free, you have dry skin. Other signs of dry skin are a tight, pinched look and small pores.

What's essential to know is that each skin type requires its own program of care. So, if you've been following a program and it hasn't been working, nine times out of 10 it's because the program isn't suited to your skin type. It's that simple.

Choose one of the following programs to help your skin look its best and most radiant now.

These programs are basic routines for the most common skin types, including sensitive skin, which is identifiable by its negative reactions to products and the environment. There are also other specific types of problem skin, for example, skin marred with deep wrinkles, sun damage, acne (see Chapter 3), rosacea, and other conditions. The products recommended here, like those I suggest my patients use, are composed of non-comedogenic (non-pore-blocking) ingredients and are, for the most part, fragrance free. I do discuss other department store and drugstore products and their characteristics in other chapters, so you need not feel confined to just the products I mention. Feel free to experiment, as long as the products you like are suitable for your skin type and you get the okay from a dermatologist.

Program for Oily Skin

When you have oily skin, your oil glands work overtime, producing more oil than you need and leaving behind an obvious sheen. To help your condition (and it is a condition):

- Wash your face twice daily with a cleanser containing an alpha hydroxy acid or a salicylic acid (such as SalAc Wash or Johnson & Johnson Clean & Clear).
- Immediately after cleansing, apply an oil-free moisturizer with sun block in the morning (such as Purpose) and an oil-free moisturizer at night (such as Neutrogena).
- Every week, give yourself a mask specifically for oily skin.
- If you're really oily and the cleansers aren't helping enough, you can try applying a low-concentration over-the-counter benzoyl peroxide product to help diminish oil production.

- You may also want to try a vitamin A topical solution or an over-the-counter or prescription-strength preparation that contains sulfur.
- In extreme cases, when you just can't seem to stop the oil from producing, you can get a prescription of low-dose Accutane, a member of the vitamin A family.

Program for Combination Skin

The main way to tell whether you have combination skin is to check for an oily T-zone area (forehead and nose) and dry cheeks. Many people with so-called combination skin actually have a medical condition called seborrheic eczema, or seborrhea, in which oil glands overproduce oils in the face and scalp, while an overproduction of yeast further stimulates oil production in those areas.

- To treat combination skin, start at the scalp. You'll need a skin-care routine that addresses both your oily and dry areas.
- Use anti-seborrheic shampoos (such as T-Sal, Head and Shoulders Intensive Treatment, or Denorex) or anti-yeast shampoos (such as Nizoral AD). After washing your hair and scalp with these medicated shampoos at least twice a week for a period of eight weeks, you'll see a marked reduction in oiliness and a rebalancing of the oily and dry areas.
- Avoid using gels and hair sprays as they can migrate down to the face and block pores.
- Wash your skin with either a non-soap cleanser (such as Cetaphil), or a salicylic cleanser (such as SalAc).
- You can further reduce oil by alternating your cleanser with a soap containing zinc pyrithione, an active ingredient that helps seborrheic dermatitis (try ZNP Bar by Steifel).
- After cleansing, always apply an oil-free moisturizer that contains a sunscreen with SPF 15.
- Use a combination of two masks on your skin once a week, applying a clay-based mask to oily areas and a moisturizing mask to dry areas.

Program for Normal Skin

Cleanse twice daily with Cetaphil Liquid cleanser or a glycolic acid cleanser like GlyDerm for extra exfoliating benefits.

- In the morning, use NeoStrata Daytime Skin Smoothing cream for the 8 percent glycolic acid and SPF 15 it contains.
- For evening, choose between or alternate products containing vitamin A, vitamin C, and plant extracts, like Neutrogena Healthy Skin Anti-Wrinkle cream, MD Forte Skin Rejuvenation Lotion,

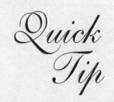

Quick Tip

If you have sensitive skin, avoid these common irritants in products: fragrance, preservatives (parabens, quaternium 15, sodium benzoate), lanolin, essential oils (on your face), alpha hydroxy acids, vitamin E, dyes, and PABA (used in some sunscreens).

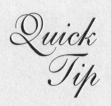

Retin-A, Retin-A Micro, and Avita (all vitamin A products). You can also use Citrix or Cellex-C (vitamin C products), and/or Kinerase. Anytime you feel the need for more moisture, you can use an oil-free moisturizer like Hydrotone Lite.

Program for Dry Skin

When you have dry skin, taking steps to make sure your skin has enough moisture should be a part of your daily routine.

* Cleanse your skin twice daily, using a liquid, moisturizing, nonsoap cleanser (such as Cetaphil, Basis, Neutrogena, Oilatum AD, or Pond's).
* After washing, apply a soothing moisturizer while the skin is still slightly moist or damp to help trap water into the skin. (For best results, always apply creams and lotions onto damp skin.)
* Make sure to use a non-greasy moisturizer. People with dry skin tend to load up their skin with creamy moisturizers. However, these heavy products can clog pores, leading to breakouts.
* Neutrogena and Purpose by Johnson & Johnson have nourishing, rich and creamy (but non-greasy), formulas that won't clog your pores and will help heal extra-dry skin, leaving you feeling smooth to the touch.
* After you've applied moisturizer, spread on a good, broad-spectrum sunscreen. Always use a sunscreen with an SPF of at least 15.
* Every week, give yourself a moisturizing mask.
* Drink plenty of water every day–eight 8-ounce glasses a day.
* Avoid washing clothing in harsh detergents, which can irritate dry, as well as sensitive, skin. Use a dye- and fragrance-free detergent. Certain detergents can be less irritating to the skin than others. If your skin is sensitive, itchy, or dry, simply changing your laundry detergent may solve the problem.

Program for Sensitive Skin

Patients constantly tell me they have sensitive skin. Most don't. How to tell: your skin reacts to almost anything. That is, if you're wearing no makeup, no moisturizer, and no sunscreen, and your skin still reacts, it's sensitive. Before doing anything, it's important to first confirm that you do have sensitive skin and not something else entirely, such as rosacea, eczema, or sun damage. If you are unsure, it's always a good idea to consult a dermatologist.

* To keep sensitive skin smooth and free of blotchiness, use products that contain as few preservatives, fragrances, and chemicals as possible.
* In the morning, wash your skin using a mild cleanser (such as Cetaphil or Oilatum AD).

- Avoid using toners on sensitive skin. Most toners contain alcohol, which can dry and irritate sensitive skin.
- Apply a light, water-based moisturizer. Look for products that are mild and hydrating. Check the label for buzzwords, such as alcohol-free, colorant-free, soap-free, fragrance-free, non-comedogenic, and non-acnegenic. Try non-greasy Lubriderm Advanced Therapy or Lubriderm Seriously Sensitive Lotion, which is lanolin-free, dye-free, and fragrance-free, to protect skin from the usual causes of irritation and breakouts. Other fragrance-free products include Curél lotion, Moisturel, and Cetaphil.
- Put on an oil-free and fragrance-free sunblock.
- Wear oil-free, hypoallergenic makeup (such as Almay or Clinique).
- You may also want to check out the type of detergent you are using. Avoid trouble by using fragrance-free and dye-free detergents (such as Cheer Free or All Free).

Typical Areas For Rosacea Symptoms

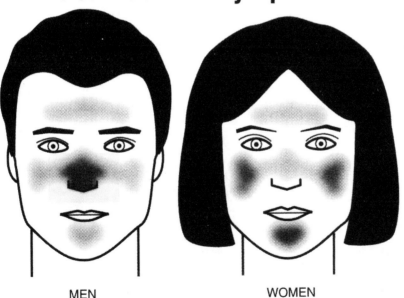

MEN   WOMEN

According to a National Rosacea Society patient survey on the pattern of rosacea symptoms, rosacea tends to affect men and women differently. Women are more likely to experience symptoms on the cheeks (87 percent of women versus 68 percent of men) and chin (49 percent of women versus 20 percent of men), while men are more likely to have swelling of the nose associated with advanced rosacea (21 percent of men versus 8 percent of women).

REPRINTED BY PERMISSION OF THE NATIONAL ROSACEA SOCIETY, BARRINGTON, IL.

Myth:

You can catch rosacea from someone else who has it.

FACT:

Rosacea is basically a genetic condition seen most commonly in light-skinned people in their thirties or forties. Someone with the condition often has red cheeks and sometimes a red nose, which may be accompanied by pus pimples and red bumps. It doesn't look great in its advanced stages, but it's certainly not contagious or catching. It also means the person's skin has sustained considerable sun damage that has broken down the collagen around the blood capillaries, causing them to dilate and increase blood flow to the skin. That is why people with rosacea have chronic redness. The increased blood flow may also be to blame for the broken capillaries and the pimples that can crop up.

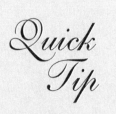

For more information and tips on rosacea, check out the National Rosacea Society's Web site at www.rosacea.org.

Program for Rosacea

If you have a rosy tinge to your cheeks and dilated blood vessels around your cheeks and your nose, you probably have rosacea. This inherited condition shows up on the face as dilated, broken blood vessels, a tendency toward flushing, and little breakouts of tiny white pustules. Spicy food, sun exposure, working out, and alcohol can aggravate rosacea. This condition predominantly affects men and women with fair complexions. Although no one knows precisely why people with lighter complexions are more prone to rosacea, experts believe fair skin tends to get more sun damage, which results in dilating blood vessels that ultimately burst. The sun also damages the collagen, which is the support structure for the blood vessels. So fair-skinned folks get a double whammy: the sun's ultraviolet rays both dilate blood vessels and damage the supporting collagen that keeps the blood vessels small and invisible inside the skin.

People with rosacea often experience facial flushing or blushing under stress. If you have rosacea, you may or may not have pimples, but you probably will have a background of redness or broken blood vessels across the main area of the cheeks (close to the nose) as well as on the nose and maybe even the chin.

Most Common Rosacea Tripwires

Percent of rosacea patients affected by the most common factors that may trigger rosacea flare-ups, based on a survey of more than 400 rosacea sufferers.

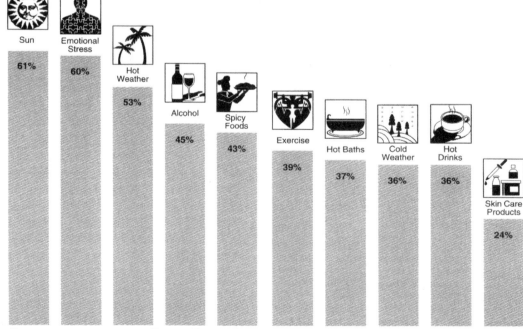

- Cleanse in the morning with a non-irritating liquid cleanser (such as Cetaphil, Oilatum AD, or Neutrogena).
- Apply an oil-free moisturizer with sunblock (such as Purpose or Oil of Olay).
- In the evening, cleanse with a non-irritating cleanser.
- Apply a prescription sulfur-containing cream (such as Novacet or Sulfacet-R).
- To stabilize and treat the condition, doctors often prescribe topical antibiotics, such as metronidazole, or oral antibiotics, such as tetracycline, minocycline, doxycycline, or erythromycin.
- Other remedies include blood pressure medications (such as Clonidine or Corgard).
- Azelex, an acne medication, is also sometimes prescribed.
- Laser treatments with the Pulsed Dye Laser are sometimes prescribed to help tone down the redness (see Chapter 14).

Program for Sun-Damaged/Wrinkled Skin

Skin that has been damaged by the sun, which is the major cause of wrinkling, needs a gentle touch. (See Chapter 12 for more on the sun and skin.) Over time, the cumulative effects of the sun's rays break down the skin's collagen and elastin, which affects the skin's elasticity and ability to bounce back (thus the sagging or wrinkling). As the skin defends itself against the damage, it gets thicker, which is why chronic sunbathers often develop facial skin that is as thick

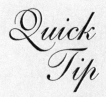

Quick Tip

If you have rosacea, you need to watch the powder and foundation you use. Many of the most popular powders now are iridescent. The iridescence (or shine) comes from ground-up mica in the formulation. The rough-edged particles of mica can over time lodge into your skin, causing irritations, breakouts, and milia (tiny little white sebaceous cysts that can't be squeezed). Use a matte finish for your powder and foundation, rather than products with mica or light-reflecting particles in them.

Foods That Can Cause Flare-Ups

Percentages of rosacea sufferers affected by specific foods and beverages that may trigger rosacea flare-ups, based on a survey of more than 3,000 sufferers affected by these factors.

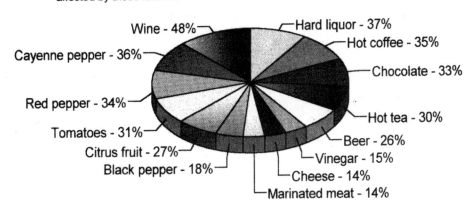

Wine - 48%
Hard liquor - 37%
Cayenne pepper - 36%
Hot coffee - 35%
Chocolate - 33%
Red pepper - 34%
Tomatoes - 31%
Hot tea - 30%
Citrus fruit - 27%
Beer - 26%
Black pepper - 18%
Vinegar - 15%
Cheese - 14%
Marinated meat - 14%

REPRINTED BY PERMISSION OF THE NATIONAL ROSACEA SOCIETY, BARRINGTON, IL.

as cowhide. Because skin that has been overexposed to the sun is already so damaged, you need to treat it more gently.

- Cleanse your face every morning with a mild, non-irritating cleanser (such as Cetaphil Liquid, Oilatum AD, fragrance-free Dove, or Neutrogena).
- Next put on a sunscreen containing alpha hydroxy acids, which will help to slough off the thickened dead skin cells.
- In the evening, wash your face with the same cleanser you used in the morning.
- Apply a vitamin A–based cream (such as Retin-A) or a cream that contains retinol (such as Neutrogena Healthy Skin Anti-Wrinkle Cream or Estée Lauder Diminish Retinol Treatment).
- You also can apply an emollient eye cream containing alpha hydroxy acid (such as Avon Anew Perfect Eye Care Cream) to help rehydrate delicate skin.
- Another antioxidant, called coenzyme Q10 (CoQ10), is a nutrient found in the human body that helps convert food into energy. This important antioxidant diminishes as we age, contributing to premature aging. You can find CoQ10 in Nivea Visage Q10 Wrinkle Control Face Creme and Nivea Q10 Wrinkle Control Eye Creme.
- Plant-based Kinerase, which you can get from your dermatologist, may also help reduce sun damage and stimulate collagen production.
- Copper is an essential element in collagen production and in forming new blood vessels. Because you may not get enough copper in your skin through your diet, you can increase the copper in your skin by applying it topically. Neova offers skin-care products with copper in them, and Osmotics, a Denver, Colorado–based company, offers a copper-based cream called Blue Copper.
- Always protect your hands, which are usually exposed to the sun continuously, with sunscreen to keep them from showing signs of aging (such as age spots and wrinkles).

Common Questions

Q: My skin is very dry, but oils don't help it. Am I doing something wrong?

A: Dry skin is actually low in water, not in oil. That's why most moisturizers list water as the first ingredient in the label. You need to realize that water, not oil, is the ingredient you need to add moisture back into the skin. Many people instead apply an occlusive product, such as Vaseline or petrolatum, onto dry skin, thinking that will do the trick and hydrate the skin. It won't, unless you first put water on the skin. Then, the product will work as a seal. If you are acne prone, however, stay away from any moisturizers containing topical oils. Instead, go for lighter, oil-free moisturizers that contain humectants, such as glycerin, to trap and hold moisture onto the skin. If you aren't acne prone, then you can pretty much use any moisturizer (even those containing oils). Whatever moisturizer you use, always apply it to slightly damp skin, so that any extra water on the skin's surface absorbs into the skin and is trapped there.

Q: I have oily skin. What kinds of products, other than benzoyl peroxide, can I use on my skin, without irritating it?

A: If you have oily skin, you can use a number of good products other than low-concentration benzoyl peroxide. Salicylic acid, which is available over the counter, is great for oily skin. So are topical vitamin A products. Other products that work to reduce oil production include over-the-counter or prescription-strength sulfur-containing preparations. In extreme cases, your dermatologist can place you on a low dose of Accutane to reduce sebaceous oil production. Remember, oily hair, because it touches your face, can lead to oily skin. So, increase the number of shampoos you give yourself each week or try a medicated shampoo (such as T-Sal, T-Gel, or Nizoral AD), and you'll find that your skin will become less oily over time.

Q: I have so many skin-care products. Is there a special order in which I'm supposed to put them on?

A: Yes—and at specific times too. In the morning after cleansing your skin, apply sunblock first because, to be effective, it needs about 30 minutes to absorb into your skin. Wait 10 to 15 minutes before applying any alpha hydroxy acid (AHA) product, so it doesn't dilute the sunscreen. Then finish up with a moisturizer. As an alternative and to save steps, you can use a moisturizer with built-in sunscreen and AHAs. Finally, if necessary, dab on any over-the-counter pimple creams. (If you're using prescription preparations, ask your doctor at what stage they should be applied.)

Quick Tip

Rosacea sufferers should make an investment in sable brushes. They are far less irritating to the skin than other applicators or brushes. Unlike sponge applicators, you can wash sable brushes. (You can even throw them in the dishwasher.) You can usually find sable brushes at high-end department stores as well as at many mass retail outlets for much less money.

If you're using any vitamin A products (Retin-A, Renova, or retinol) or vitamin C serums (Cellex-C), use them before bedtime. If you use both A and C products, apply them on alternating nights; when used together, they can cancel each other out. You should apply vitamin A products 20 to 30 minutes before you go to sleep, because unabsorbed cream can smear on your pillow and irritate eyes. Moisturizer can go on immediately after the vitamins.

chapter two

The United Nations of Skin Care

Beauty is in the eye of the beholder.
—PROVERB

EACH ETHNIC SKIN TYPE—CAUCASIAN, ASIAN, LATINO, AMERICAN-INDIAN, AND Arab, African, or Indo-European—comes with its own specific set of problems and treatments. In this chapter, several of my colleagues who specialize in ethnic skin offer their words of advice on how to handle the unique challenges of these skin types, as follows:

Latino Skin: Covered by Maritza I. Perez, M.D., dermatologist at The Center for Dermatology, Cosmetic and Laser Surgery, Mount Kisco, New York, and Associate Clinical Professor of Dermatolgy at Columbia University, New York
Black Skin: Covered by Susan C. Taylor, M.D., director of the Skin of Color Center at St. Luke's Roosevelt University Hospital, New York, New York
Asian Skin: Covered by Grace H. Pak, M.D., dermatologist at The Center for Dermatology, Cosmetic and Laser Surgery, Mount Kisco, New York

Latino Skin

Latino skin gets its appearance and characteristics from a genetic background that might include Spanish, Northern and Southern American Indian, and African heritage. German, Italian, and/or Portuguese influences are also sometimes present in this skin type.

Because of the variable genetics of this skin type, Latino skin varies in its sensitivity to the sun. For example, Latino skin that includes American Indian influences (brown, smooth-textured skin, not acne prone, with straight dark hair) does not burn as easily as Latino skin with a predominantly Caucasian genetic background. Men

11

and women who have more of a bronze tone to their skin often tan before burning and can have problems with pigmentation. If the skin is mainly black in color, it may be prone to acne.

How to Treat Sun Damage in...

Light Latino Skin

Latinos with light skin suffer from cumulative sun damage, so it gets worse as the person ages. (See Table 1, skin types III and IV.) To heal and protect this type of skin, it is helpful to use bleaching creams, Azelex, and sunblocks with a high SPF.

Bronze Latino Skin

Latinos with a bronze-tone skin color tend to have delicate skin features, most likely inherited from an American Indian ancestry. This skin type tends to get deeper pigmentation, even with minimal sun exposure (see Table 1, skin types IV and V). A hormonal component of this skin type makes it more likely to get hyperpigmentation, patches of darker, uneven color all over the skin. Early intervention requires regular use of bleaching creams as well as high-SPF, chemical-free sunblocks. Since bronze Latino skin is more sensitive to irritants, I suggest using beta hydroxy acids rather than alpha hydroxy acids, because beta hydroxy acids are milder.

Very Dark Latino Skin

Latinos with this skin type respond to the sun in the same way African Americans do. Hyperpigmentation (unevenness and blotchy dark patches) is their major skin problem. Bleaching creams and Azelex can help with this problem.

Program for Latino Skin

- Wash with a gentle cleanser twice daily.
- Apply sunscreen daily, no matter how dark or light your skin tone is.
- In the morning, apply a glycolic acid moisturizer.
- In the evening, alternate an application of adapelene (Differin) with an application of vitamin C.
- Get glycolic acid, amino fruit acid, or beta hydroxy acid peels, if possible, which can be very helpful in maintaining a smooth skin texture and youthful glow.
- As skin ages, switch from adapelene to tretinoin (Retin-A) at night and add lightening gels to help erase blotchy dark patches.
- For older skin, you can also increase the strength of the office treatments and consider TCA or Jessner/Efudex peels. (Read about these peels in Chapter 11.)

- To take care of deeper wrinkles, consider using the erbium:YAG laser, superficial dermabrasion, and/or a face-lift.

Black Skin

The major biological factor that separates black skin from white skin is the pigment melanin. Although people with black skin and with white skin have the same number of pigment-producing cells, called melanocytes, the melanocytes in black skin produce significantly more pigment, making it darker. Scientists estimate there are 35 hues, or shades, of black skin; there are probably several more shades than that. Most Black women living in America today probably descend from a combination of African as well as American Indian, Asian, and/or European ancestors. These combinations can produce an endless array of skin tones, facial features, and hair textures among dark-skinned people.

How to Treat Sun Damage in Black Skin

One terrific advantage of having large amounts of melanin in the skin is that the melanin protects black skin from the sun and from many of the ravages of sun-induced aging. Luckily, Black women are also less susceptible to developing skin cancer, especially basal cell carcinoma and squamous cell carcinoma, because the melanin in their skin acts as protection. (See Table 1, group VI for darker tones and group V for light-skinned Blacks.) Nevertheless, a sunscreen with an SPF of 15 to 30 should be applied daily to help protect against getting dark blotches from exposure to sunlight. It will also help fade dark blemishes on black skin. Bleaching creams and Azelex can also be used to help bleach dark blotches on sun-damaged skin.

Program for Black Skin

- Cleanse the skin gently twice a day, using fingertips (not a washcloth) and a mild, nonirritating cleanser. Carefully pat the skin dry.
- Avoid using cleansers that contain abrasive granules, which can irritate the skin and break capillaries. Also avoid using acne puffs and rough washcloths.
- Apply moisturizer to the face if it is dry, ashen, or taut after cleansing.
- Every day apply a sunscreen with an SPF of 15 to 30 to protect against damaging UV rays and to fade any dark blemishes you already have.

Common Skin Problems

Black skin can be affected by several fairly common skin conditions, which follow, as well as by another less common condition, vitiligo.

Problem: Acne eruptions

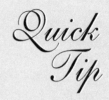

Quick Tip

Many women with black skin have a natural sun protection factor of 13 (SPF 13). So, with fewer wrinkles and age spots, Black women may look up to 10 or 15 years younger than do Caucasian, Asian, or Latino women of the same age.

Solution: With black skin, any rash must be treated quickly to avoid the possibility of abnormal pigmentation. Similarly, you should treat all acne eruptions quickly, and you should avoid picking, squeezing, or manipulating the bumps. It is also important to see a dermatologist if pigment problems develop.

Problem: Discoloration of elbows and knees (darker than surrounding skin)
Solution:
* Avoid all trauma to the area, including leaning on the elbows or kneeling.
* Apply a hydroquinone bleaching cream or Azelex to the areas every morning and again at night. If over-the-counter products are not working well enough, you may need to see a dermatologist for a stronger, prescription hydroquinone product.
* Exfoliate the areas daily, using an alpha hydroxy acid product.

Problem: Small or large brown growths on the face and neck
Solution: A dermatologist can easily remove these bumps—which are hereditary, benign, and will not become cancerous. No cream or lotion will take them away or prevent them from appearing.

Problem: Any type of pimple, acne, rash, or inflammation of the skin produces dark marks or patches, termed postinflammatory hyperpigmentation, which may take months or even years to fade. The loss of pigment is not as serious as in vitiligo (wherein the melanin disappears from the skin, and white patches appear). Still, it may take a long while for the skin color to fade or blend in with the normal surrounding skin.
Solution: Apply bleaching creams containing hydroquinone as well as Azelex.

Problem: Melasma, or dark patches on the cheeks and forehead, is another pigmentation disorder common to black-skinned people. It is particularly common in women who take oral contraceptives or who are pregnant. Exposure to the sun makes melasma worse and can prevent melasma from fading.
Solution: Melasma usually responds to the topical application of hydroquinone bleaching agents, Azelex, sunscreens, and chemical peels.

Problem: Keloids, large and unsightly scars, form during the healing process of a wound when the body continues to uncontrollably produce large amounts of scar tissue after the injury is healed. Although keloids may occur anywhere on the body, they occur most commonly on the earlobes, chest, and back.

Solution: Prevention, if possible, or three available treatments.

- Most dermatologists shrink a keloid by injecting it several times with either a cortisone solution or a medication called interferon.
- Dermatologists sometimes remove keloids with laser surgery or scar revision surgery (actually cutting out the scar). However, the keloid may recur, especially if the area was not injected with cortisone immediately following the surgery.
- Some cosmetic surgeons recommend Mederma, an over-the-counter cream, either to improve existing scars or to prevent scars from forming during the healing process.
- The best treatment is prevention by avoiding all unnecessary surgery and body piercing. Unfortunately, if you have one keloid, chances are high you will develop more.

Problem: Vitiligo, a disease in which the melanin (pigment) disappears from the skin and white patches appear, appears less frequently than the other skin problems covered in this chapter. Vitiligo can be psychologically devastating.

Solution: Pigment can be restored with topical creams or special ultraviolet light treatments. Support groups are available to help sufferers overcome the psychological effects of vitiligo.

Unique Characteristics of Normal Black Skin
Certain features are normal in healthy black skin, including:

Futcher's Lines: A line on the upper arm, which separates the lighter skin on the inside of the arm from the darker skin tone on the outside.

Mid-line Hypopigmentation: A genetic condition in which the skin on the middle of the chest is lighter in color than the skin toward the side.

Hyperpigmented Keratotic Palmar Pitting: Small pinpoint holes in the palms, some of which may have a thickened, darkly colored core.

Palmar Crease Hyperpigmentation: Darkened creases in the palm.

Gingival Hyperpigmentation: Darkened gums around the teeth.

Pigmented Nail Streaks: Dark brown streaks on the nails, running from end to end.

A word of caution: If only one nail has this streak, it could be a sign of a serious type of skin cancer that requires an immediate examination and biopsy by a dermatologist.

Camouflaging Moves for Black Skin
If you have uneven pigmentation, you can camouflage the dark patches with concealer and foundation. Follow these steps:

Myth:

Leave your scrapes uncovered so they will heal.

FACT:

Contrary to what your grandmother may have told you, wounds prefer a closed, moist environment in which to heal. Keeping a scrape or cut covered with a bandage and antibiotic ointment is the quickest way to healing with the least chance of leaving a scar or mark.

- Choose a concealer that is one or two shades lighter than your normal skin.
- Make sure the concealer is creamy, not thick or chalky.
- After patting a thin layer of concealer directly on the dark area, blend in carefully into the surrounding area, and set with face powder.
- Cover the areas you've concealed with foundation that matches your normal skin tone. After applying, look at it indoors as well as outdoors in daylight to make sure it's the right color. The undertone of the product (yellow, red, or orange) should match the undertone of your natural skin color.
- Dust over the foundation with face powder.

Asian Skin

Asian skin is normally yellow in color, but the tone can vary, depending on the region the man or woman comes from. The yellow skin color is usually the result of a high amount of melanin. Asians seem to have a lower incidence of skin cancer than Caucasians do.

How to Treat Sun Damage in Asian Skin

The increased amount of thickness and melanin found in most Asian skin provides a natural form of protection against sun damage. Still, Asian skin is prone to melasma (dark patches), freckles, and age spots (see Table 1, group V). To protect and heal Asian skin, it's important to use a sunscreen with a minimum SPF 15. A vitamin A derivative product (such as Retin-A, Renova, or retinol) can also help reverse the effects of sun damage.

Program for Asian Skin

- Each morning use a gentle cleanser.
- After cleansing, apply a moisturizer that contains a pigment-controlling ingredient, such as hydroquinone (such as Porcelana or Lustra AF), azeleic acid (such as Azelex), or kojic acid (such as products from Physicians' Choice of Arizona).
- Every day apply a broad-spectrum sunscreen with a minimum SPF 15 to protect skin from the melasma (dark patches), freckles, and age spots to which Asian skin is prone.
- In the evening, use a gentle cleanser and one or more of the "rejuvenating" family of products: retinoids (such as Retin-A, Renova, or retinol), alpha hydroxy acids (glycolic acid), beta hydroxy acids (salicylic acid), antioxidants (vitamin C), or Kinerase.
- Asian skin can benefit from superficial laser resurfacing to erase fine lines, acne, melasma, and mild photodamage.

- Light chemical peels (glycolic, amino fruit acid, and beta hydroxy acid) and microdermabrasion (particle resurfacing) can help keep Asian skin smooth and glowing.
- Asian skin tends to be more sensitive to alpha hydroxy acids than to beta hydroxy acids.
- Laser resurfacing, deeper peels, or dermabrasion can help erase deep wrinkles, acne scarring, and moderate to severe sun damage. In most cases, the high risk of pigment changes and scarring makes Asians poor candidates for laser resurfacing; however, the procedure sometimes works if proper skin-care and sun-protection routines are regularly followed.

Botanical Skin Lighteners for Asian Skin

- Kojic acid has become a popular bleaching agent, because many Asians are unable to tolerate hydroquinone.
- Mulberry extracts, chamomile, licorice extract and arbutin (a plant based ingredient) have been shown to exhibit some skin lightening effects.
- Mushroom extract and Asian turnip extract have been used in several skin-lightening powders sold in Asia.
- Rice powder, rice made into a paste by grounding it down into a powder and adding water to it, also is known to inhibit tyrosinase. Rice extract contains a high concentration of PABA, a very effective sunscreen, as well as ferulic acid and allantoin, both of which are also sunscreens.

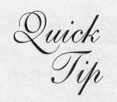

Quick Tip

Botanical extracts, such as coffee oil, algae extract, and pearl extract, filter UV light well, adding a boost to skin-lightening products.

TABLE 1
FITZPATRICK CHART
SKIN TYPES AND THEIR REACTIONS TO SUNLIGHT

SKIN TYPE	UNEXPOSED SKIN COLOR	SENSITIVITY	SUNBURN AND TANNING HISTORY
I	White	Very Sensitive	Burns easily, never tans. Usually red hair, green eyes, freckles.
II	White	Very Sensitive	Burns easily, tans minimally with difficulty. Typically blond hair, blue eyes.
III	White	Sensitive	Burns minimally; tans gradually and uniformly (light brown). Generally brown hair, blue or hazel eyes.
IV	Light brown	Moderately Sensitive	Burns minimally; always tans well (moderate brown). Usually brown hair, brown eyes, olive complexion.
V	Brown	Minimally Sensitive	Rarely burns; tans profusely (dark brown). Most Asians, Latinos, American Indians, and light-skinned Blacks.
VI	Dark-brown or Black	Least Sensitive; Insensitive	Never burns; tans profusely; deeply (black). Most dark-skinned Blacks and Australian Aborigines.

chapter three

About Face

An ounce of prevention is worth a pound of cure.
—Proverb

Best Way to Wash Your Face

Knowing the proper cleansing routine and your best maintenance beauty level won't benefit you if you don't understand the best technique by which to get there. In other words, there is a right way and a wrong way to wash your face, exfoliate your face, apply moisturizer, and apply a mask. It doesn't matter how much correct information I've provided you with, if you do the techniques wrong, you won't get the results you want. So, let's start with the best way to wash your face.

The best way to wash your face is to use warm water and a mild cleanser twice a day, probably in the morning and then before you go to bed. It sounds simple, but like most things in life, it's all in the details. Here's the step-by-step process:

1. Place a small pool of cleanser on your palm.
2. Using your fingertips, gently rub the cleanser all over your face for 15 to 30 seconds.
3. Splash your face with running warm water several times (about 10), until you feel that all the cleanser has rinsed off. Feel your face for signs of oily residue.
4. Pat your face slightly with a clean face towel, but make sure not to pat completely dry—you need some water to remain on the skin.
5. Apply moisturizer by dotting it all over your face and blending it in thoroughly.

Cleansing Thoughts

Choosing the right cleanser, like choosing a moisturizer and a mask, is determined by your skin type. You might also need to consider the time of the year, because your skin typically changes with the seasons. Usually, skin gets oilier in the summer and drier in the winter, so you'll probably want to change your cleanser from season to season.

Think about what you truly need in a cleanser. Do you want something anti-bacterial? You do, if you are cleansing skin that is acne- or eczema-prone. However, don't stress too much over your cleanser. It goes on the skin for less than a minute with each cleansing, twice a day, as opposed to moisturizer or night cream, which lay on the skin for eight hours or more. Figure out the rest of your routine first, then choose a cleanser, rather than the other way around. Makes sense, doesn't it?

Go to the Cleaners

Here are a few examples of inexpensive cleansers that I highly recommend:

Cetaphil Anti-bacterial Bar
Basis cleanser
Cetaphil Liquid cleanser
Oilatum AD (anti-bacterial)
Fragrance-free Dove for sensitive skin
Purpose cleanser
Neutrogena bar and liquid cleansers
Oil of Olay Daily Renewal Cleanser

If your skin is particularly acne-prone, aim for cleansers that contain either benzoyl peroxide or salicylic acid. By the way, when it comes time to splash your face with water, I recommend following one of my favorite sayings: "Everything in moderation." Not too cold, not too hot, not too much, not too little. Neither extreme cold nor hot water is good for your face (despite what Joan Crawford said about dunking her face in a bowl of ice water or ice cubes). Both extremes in temperature are sure to break delicate blood vessels and capillaries. As I said, it is better to rinse your face every time using warm or tepid water.

Best Way to Exfoliate Your Face

Did you know that your skin sheds its dead skin cells on a daily basis (in fact, each time you vacuum, you're picking up dead skin cells off the floor, the chair, the wall, etc.). It's true. In fact, even while you sleep, mother nature is doing her job by making sure your skin exfoliates itself, without your help.

Still, some days (or nights) you want to glow as much as possible. For those times, I recommend you exfoliate. Men don't need to worry as much about exfoliating, because they do it every time they use a razor to shave. Here's the best way to exfoliate your face:

1. Take a little bit of the exfoliating cream or gel specifically for your skin type and gently rub it onto your already cleansed face.
2. Lightly rub the mixture around your nose, cheeks, and chin, where skin tends to become irritated when pores are clogged. Rub for only about 10 seconds to avoid irritation.
3. Rinse with warm water, until you feel no more grains.
4. Pat slightly with a towel.
5. Apply moisturizer.

Puff Stuff

One thing I tell my patients is, depending on their skin type, using products or devices such as loofahs, buff puffs, and washcloths may prove too irritating to the skin. Another reason I discourage using these products is that they can easily become a fertile ground for bacterial growth (after all, how many of us really wash out these things)? What really happens is the loofah, buff puff, or washcloth ends up sitting around gathering bacteria. It also usually stays in the shower, and damp, creating a perfect breeding ground on which bacteria can grow. Then, you pick up this bacteria-laden scrubber and rub it into your face. This is a recipe for disaster. A few days or even hours later you can develop a severe skin irritation or rash, possibly leading to an infection. That's why I don't advocate exfoliating for every skin type, although it usually is helpful for people with oily skin. As I've mentioned before, our skin exfoliates itself naturally. If it didn't, we'd all weigh 800 pounds!

Toning Talk

Despite what you've read or what a department store cosmetologist has told you in order to sell you one more product you don't need, applying toner is not always a necessary part of a skin-care routine. The only exception is oily skin, which may need that extra step of toning to make it feel squeaky clean (especially if your face feels sticky or oily even after washing it). Otherwise, it's wise to be wary of using toner. Most toners contain alcohol or witch hazel, both of which are drying to the skin and especially irritating to dry or sensitive skin. Don't be fooled into thinking that it's okay to use witch hazel as a toner because it doesn't contain alcohol; it still dries out the skin. You may want to go with an alcohol-free toner that has a main ingredient of chamomile or rose water, both of which are soothing to the skin.

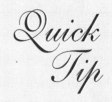

Quick Tip

Have you somehow exfoliated your face until it's raw? Soothe the irritation and reduce the redness by washing with a gentle soap (like Cetaphil) and spreading a thin layer of 1 percent cortisone cream over the chafed areas.

Best Moisturizers

If you've ever wondered "which moisturizer is right for me," you're not alone. Moisturizers make up a $1 billion market in the United States, but because of the vast array of products available, selecting a moisturizer can be confusing. If you choose the wrong moisturizer, your skin can suffer–more so than if you select the wrong cleanser, exfoliator, or mask. The reason: moisturizer sits on your skin for the longest time, giving it ample opportunity to do real damage. For example, if you have sensitive skin but use a moisturizer formulated with a thicker, more occlusive texture, it can block your pores, irritate your face, and ultimately make your skin look worse.

There are several types of moisturizers, or humectants.

Occlusive Moisturizers

These moisturizers prevent water loss. They are oily substances that "sit" on the skin's surface and prevent evaporation through the skin. Petrolatum (or Vaseline), mineral oil, vegetable oil, and silicone are occlusive substances. Remember: dry skin lacks water, not oil, so most occlusive substances don't moisturize dry skin.

Benefits: Very few, unless applied to hydrated skin. I usually don't recommend these products, because they can clog pores. I can't tell you how many times patients have come to me complaining they have irritated, broken-out skin, and when I ask what moisturizer they've been using, they mention a petrolatum-based product.

Recommended products: Aquaphor and Eucerin moisturizing cream.

Water-in-Oil Emulsions

These formulations contain tiny droplets of water dispersed in oil, which acts as an emulsifying agent and provides a thicker barrier for dry skin. The oil is on the outside of each molecule, surrounding water, so that when you put the emulsion on your skin, you feel the oil first.

Benefits: Women over the age of 45, whose skin tends to be drier, may find that oil-based moisturizers work best, because they are thicker and richer than oil-free products. However, the trade-off is that the heavy texture of the products may block pores.

Recommended products: Nivea Creme Moisturizer and Nivea Extra-Enriched Lotion.

Oil-in-Water Emulsions

These formulations contain tiny droplets of oil dispersed in water with the help of an emulsifying agent. When these moisturizers are properly applied to the skin in a thin layer, the oil and water combine and vanish into the skin. The oil lies on the inside of each molecule, surrounded by water, so that when you put on the emulsion, you feel the water first.

Benefits: These moisturizers are more dry and less greasy on your skin than water-in-oil emulsions. For best results, you should apply oil-in-water products while the skin is still moist, such as after cleansing the skin, or when used on the body, after a bath or shower.

Recommended products: Keri Lotion and Moisturel lotion, Lubriderm lotion.

Oil-Free Moisturizers

Oil-free moisturizers contain humectants, such as propylene glycol, AHAs, or glycerin, that work like oil to help seal water into your skin.

Benefits: Though they're not quite as thick and rich as oils, these humectants will effectively hydrate your skin. They work especially well if you're prone to acne or tend to get breakouts during your menstrual cycle, because many oil-enriched products may occlude (block up) pores, leading to zits.

Recommended products: Purpose, Neutrogena Facial Moisturizer with SPF, Oil of Olay Protective Renewal Lotion, Complex 15, Purpose Alpha Hydroxy Moisture Lotion with SPF (oxybenzone), Alpha Hydrox AHA Sensitive Skin Crème (5 percent glycolic acid, oil-free), Neutrogena Healthy Skin Anti Wrinkle Cream (SPF 15, retinol, vitamin E), and Neutrogena Healthy Skin Face Lotion (SPF 15, glycolic acid, retinyl palmitate, vitamins C and E).

Vitamin-Enriched Moisturizers

Vitamin A and its derivative tretinoin (found in Retin-A, Renova, and Avita) unblock pores and reduce sun damage. Vitamin C has been shown to help prevent wrinkles and skin cancers. Vitamin E may enhance C's effects.

Benefits: Most women can benefit from vitamin-enriched products. Vitamin A can be drying, so you may be unable to use it nightly. Vitamin C becomes inactivated–that is, it breaks down–when combined with either vitamin A–containing products or AHAs. You might consider alternating your vitamin A–containing product one night and vitamin C the next night. You also need to watch out for products promoting what I call "alphabet soup," a whole host of "natural ingredients" that may add a whole lot of cost to the product with no proven benefit.

Recommended products: With vitamin C: Cellex-C, Citrix, University Medical Facelift Vitamin C- Anti-Wrinkle Patch, Sudden Change Line and Wrinkle Patches (one type with antioxidant vitamins C, E, and A, and one type with alpha hydroxy acid patches), and Neutrogena Healthy Skin Face Lotion (SPF 15, glycolic acid, retinyl palmitate, vitamins C and E).

With vitamin A: MD Forte Skin Rejuvenation Lotion I, Nivea Visage–Coenzyme Q10 Wrinkle Control Night Cream (coenzyme Q10 and retinyl palmitate), L'Oréal Plenitude Revitalift Oil-Free Lotion (retinyl palmitate), Pond's Age Defying Complex with Sunscreen (glycolic acid, retinyl palmitate,

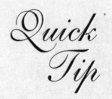

Quick Tip

Need a quick lift before a party or a special night out? Take a clean washcloth and soak it in cold water or milk from the refrigerator. Milk especially has soothing, anti-inflammatory properties. Place the compress over your eyes, and keep your head elevated so gravity will help pull extra fluid down away from your face. The cold will help constrict capillaries, which reduces redness and swelling.

Did you know that...

Your body creates a new layer of skin every 28 days.

retinyl acetate, vitamin E), Neutrogena Healthy Skin Anti Wrinkle Cream (SPF 15, retinol, vitamin E), and Oil of Olay ProVital Night Cream (retinyl palmitate and vitamin E).

Alpha Hydroxy Acids

AHAs hydrate the skin, exfoliate the skin, revitalize sun-damaged skin, and open pores.

Benefits: They slough off the top, dead skin-cell layer, leaving skin glowing and reducing acne. Anyone can use them if you find the formulation that suits you best. Oily skin? Then opt for a lotion. If your skin tends to be drier, you may opt for a cream. Don't overuse AHAs, or your skin will react by getting red and itchy. If you get a reaction, try using a beta hydroxy acid (BHA), which is slightly milder but lacks the properties that fight sun damage.

Recommended products: Neutrogena Healthy Skin Face Lotion (SPF 15, glycolic acid, retinyl palmitate, vitamins C and E), Alpha Hydrox AHA Sensitive Skin Crème (5 percent glycolic acid, oil-free), Purpose Alpha Hydroxy Moisture Lotion with SPF (oxybenzone), Neutrogena Multivitamin Acne Treatment (salicylic acid, vitamins A and E, glycolic acid), and Neostrata Skin Smoothing Cream.

Spray-On Mists

Composed mostly of water, these mists instantly hydrate the skin.

Benefits: When used alone, a mist adds only a little moisture, but if you follow it with a cream or lotion, you instantly seal in the moisture on dry skin. Another plus: mists are portable, mess-free, and user-friendly.

Recommended products: Almay Stress Tonic and Evian.

Best Way to Moisturize

Your skin type dictates the amount and type of moisturizer you need. Like cleansers, your choice of moisturizer may change as the seasons change. In fact, in the summer most people need a lighter moisturizer and will change back to a heavier, richer moisturizer around wintertime.

Choosing the right moisturizer is key to taking care of your skin and looking great, and it's very important to figure out what type of moisturizer is best for your skin type. To do this, ask yourself a few questions:

Are you prone to acne, pimples, breakouts, or blocked pores? If you are, realize that recent studies indicate that 40 to 50 percent of adults between the ages of 20 and 40 are diagnosed with persistent, low-grade acne. If you are one of these people, then you will want to use oil-free moisturizing products (see above). I recommend that women with these skin problems choose products that contain glycolic acid or another alpha hydroxy acid. This provides a double benefit: the alpha hydroxy acid opens pores as it sloughs off dead skin cells, while it simultaneously moisturizes the skin.

When possible, you should choose a morning moisturizer that contains an SPF 15 or higher sunscreen. Some examples of oil-free moisturizers with SPF that contain an alpha hydroxy acid include products from NeoStrata, Neutrogena, and Purpose by Johnson & Johnson.

Don't neglect your neck. The neck is extremely vulnerable to lines and sagging, because the skin there contains fewer oil glands than the skin on your face, making it drier and more prone to wrinkling.

If you aren't prone to breakouts, then you can opt for basically any kind of moisturizer. If you want to save money and avoid paying for fancy packaging, you can choose from a whole array of inexpensive products, such as Lubriderm, Moisturel, fragrance-free Curél, and Eucerin.

Moisturizers work best when applied to slightly damp skin. Follow these steps for the perfect way to moisturize:

1. Cleanse, and/or exfoliate skin.
2. Pat slightly with a towel.
3. Dot moisturizer all over face and blend in thoroughly. Applying moisturizer onto a damp face helps "lock" in the water in the upper layers of the skin, preventing its evaporation. No matter what your skin type is, the best way to apply moisturizer is with your hands on slightly damp skin, because it helps lock in the water in the upper layers of the skin, sealing it onto the skin. This is a far more effective way to hydrate your skin than is simply applying moisturizer to dry skin. If your skin is slightly oily, you may need to apply moisturizer only once a day; but drier-skinned folks need to reapply several times throughout the day.

Eye Creams/Gels

To keep the delicate eye area from getting dry and "crepey," you should make it a regular part of your routine to apply a light eye gel or cream to this region. Keep the eye formula in the refrigerator for an anytime cooling treat. Avoid too heavy creams, which can clog pores. Some eye gels are firming, and when applied before your makeup, provide a temporary fix for puffy bags and wrinkles. They work by briefly trapping moisture in the uppermost skin layers. This plumps out minor lines, giving the skin a temporarily smoother appearance. Some eye creams contain caffeine and a chamomile extract, called bisabolol, that constricts capillaries and reduces swelling. Look for formulas with firming agents, such as alpha hydroxy acids, vitamin A, and vitamin C, to keep the skin taut. Look for ones that are botanically based (less irritating to sensitive skin). Comfrey and cucumber soothe and reduce swelling.

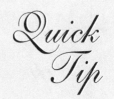

Here's a product roll call:

If you have acne, keep this in mind. The most greasy products of all are the ointments and petrolatum products. Next are creams, then gels, and then liquids. Liquids are the most drying, because they have a high alcohol content—they hit the skin and then evaporate.

Quick Tip

A great way to reap the benefits of your mask is to incorporate a gentle massage into your ritual. Here's what to do:

- First, gently cleanse your face using a circular motion and pressing lightly with the pads of the fingertips.
- Next, work your fingers out from the center of your forehead to either side of your brow.
- Massage the area under your chin, moving upward along your jawline up to your temples.
- End the massage by pressing into the area on your nose in between your eyes and by again massaging below the chin, following your jawline up to your temples.

Best Way to Apply Eye Gel/Cream

1. Always apply with your ring finger; this will keep you from applying too much pressure on the delicate skin around the eyes.
2. Pat lightly from the outer corner of the eye toward the nose.

Unmasking Masks

Masks, in my opinion, are not truly essential for all skin types. Why? Because the skin exfoliates itself 24 hours a day. Still many women like giving themselves masks and love the way their skin looks and feels afterward. So, I'm not adverse to this beauty indulgence, as long as the products are sound and do not irritate your skin. Basically, masks work as a delivery system with concentrated active ingredients, consequently achieving a more dramatic result in a shorter period of time than by either exfoliating, rehydrating, or deep cleansing the skin. Masks come in many formulations for all skin types; if you're going to use a mask, carefully select one that's right for your complexion. Here is a brief rundown of terms:

Oily Skin: Gets balanced by the oil-absorbing effects of a clay or mud mask.
Dry Skin: Gets a boost of moisture from creamy masks.
Sensitive Skin: Gets refreshed and rehydrated by light gel masks.
Combination Skin: You may need more than one mask to spot-treat different problems. To balance combination skin, for example, zap the T-zone with a deep-cleansing mask and soften cheeks and temples with a moisture-rich mask.

Best Way to Apply a Mask

1. Cleanse skin.
2. With your fingertips, apply the mask all over your face, spreading a thin layer of product evenly around. The right way to apply a mask is to pat it on gently–avoid pulling or stretching delicate facial skin as you apply the product. Don't apply it right underneath eyes; keep some space under each eye as well as around your mouth.
3. Read the package instructions for how long you should leave on the mask. A basic rule of thumb is 10 to 15 minutes, or until the mask gets hard. However, if it is a tightening mask, don't wait until it feels absolutely uncomfortable before you remove it–you'll stress your skin unnecessarily. And don't use the mask more often than once a week. Many of my patients have experienced redness and irritation from overusing their masks. I tell them that, unlike a serum or a moisturizer, a mask should be used sparingly, and it should not be kept on until it hurts.

4. Depending on the type of mask, either peel it off or rinse it off using tepid water and a washcloth.
5. Moisturize if the mask was a drying kind; otherwise hold off on the moisturizer (the mask is hydrating enough).

Bask in a Mask

Here are specific masks for each skin type and the ingredients you should look for in them:

Oily/Blemish-Prone Skin

These masks tend to contain ingredients that absorb excess oil and refine the skin's texture. Look for a clay-based (or kaolin) mask that sets on the skin. Other ingredients to look for are magnesium and sulfur, minerals that soak up oil. An exfoliating mask–especially one made with salicylic acid, a beta hydroxy acid, is anti-inflammatory (it's actually related to aspirin) and is wonderful for oily skin. Another benefit to popular alpha hydroxy masks: many of the enzymes in these masks, such as papain (from papaya) and bromelain (from pineapple), help to eat up the glue that holds the dead cells to the skin.

Recommended products: Alpha Hydrox Purifying Clay Masque (4 percent alpha hydroxy acid, kaolin and lactic acid), Neutrogena Oil Absorbing Acne Mask (5 percent benzoyl peroxide), and Bioré Self-Heating Mask (pore cleansing with kaolin and acrylates).

Dry Skin

A mask for dry skin needs to add moisture (water) to the skin's surface and seal it there. Often a gel mask provides a barrier that lets skin hang onto its own natural moisture resources. It works by using humectants that take water molecules and drag them to the skin surface, where they trap and hold the moisture in the skin. Some ingredients to look for include propylene glycol and botanical extracts like elderflower, watercress, sage, chamomile, and aloe vera.

Recommended products: Naturistics Moisturizing Facial Mask Papaya (apricot kernel oil, persimmon includes and elderflower extracts) and Bioré Self-Healing Moisture Mask (oil free).

Dry, Sun-Damaged Skin

Dry, sun-damaged skin needs a cream-based mask that's oily in consistency. The mask should be packed with ingredients that turn around the skin, such as antioxidants like vitamins A, C, and E, which help neutralize skin-damaging free radicals. Another boost can be added from alpha hydroxy acids, which can rejuvenate the skin.

Did you know that...

Clay, which is used in many beauty and spa treatments, was first discovered as a beauty ingredient by ancient Egyptian women while washing their clothes on the banks of the river Nile.

Recommended products: Naturistics Purifying Facial Mask in Sea Kelp and University Medical Face Lift Deep Wrinkle Mask.

Rewards of Retin-A

If your skin has fine, superficial lines and wrinkles, you're best served by getting a prescription for Retin-A, a topical, vitamin A derivative that can turn back the clock by stimulating collagen production in the deeper layers of the skin. Retin-A works wonderfully on sun-damaged skin and shows results in just three to six months. By stimulating the skin's collagen, it restores resiliency to aging or sun-damaged skin and promotes a faster turnover of cells. It also increases production of tiny blood vessels, which give the skin a healthy, rosy, younger look. The only downside to this wonder drug, and it's not much of one, is that you must use it daily—once you suspend use, the antiaging benefits stop as well. Since Retin-A makes skin extra-sensitive to the sun, you must also make sure to wear an SPF 15 sunscreen every day. A few people (very few) can't use Retin-A because it makes their skin ultra-dry, flaky, irritated, and supersensitive. For those people, they can try any one of the vitamin A derivatives, which are gentler on skin, such as Avita, Renova, and retinol (see Chapter 12).

Common Questions

Q: I love the way my skin looks so smooth after I exfoliate with alpha hydroxy products, but does it make me more susceptible to getting a sunburn?

A: Yes. AHA products increase your skin's sensitivity to the sun, because they thin the top layer of the epidermis. This thinning is only temporary; it lasts about three months until the skin adjusts. So, make sure to use sunscreen of SPF 15 or more.

Q: Should I use alcohol or witch hazel on my pimples?

A: Neither. Alcohol and witch hazel as well as any alcohol-based astringents actually strip away protective surface oils and irritate glands into producing more oils, which can clog pores and create unsightly blemishes.

Q: Tell me the truth about skin-care patches.

A: First, there were chemical patches to control nicotine cravings and to balance hormones. Now, dermal devices reportedly treat acne and wrinkles. These patches work like a bandage treated with an antibacterial cream. Because the patch won't slide off or evaporate, it increases the effectiveness. But here's the scoop: many creams contain the same ingredients as patches and are less cumbersome to use. However, if you want to zap a zit quickly or improve the appearance of fine lines in no time, patches can be extremely effective.

Recommended products: Bioré Fine Line Gel Patches, University Medical Facelift Vitamin C Anti-Wrinkle Patch, or BioSomme Acne Healing Patch.

Q: Should I use cold water to close my pores?

A: No. Cold water doesn't close pores and can irritate skin. In fact, there are no muscles around the pore walls, so they can't open and close. Pores remain the same size. Pores look bigger to the eye only because dead skin cells, dirt, and oil are trapped within each pore. To make the size of the pores less noticeable, rinse with cool water (which makes skin feel tighter) but not with cold water. By the same token, hot water doesn't open up pores. Warm water (not hot, which is to irritating to skin) hydrates the skin, making it easier to squeeze out dirt and debris.

Q: Is it true that if you get enough sleep, the dark circles under your eyes will disappear?

A: Unfortunately, it is not. Dark circles are hereditary. Getting enough sleep won't make circles disappear; however, not getting 40 winks will make them worse. (Skin looks more pale after a sleepless night, making circles appear darker.)

Dot the under-eye area with a yellow-based concealer (yellow neutralizes violet). Apply concealer only on the dark circle and follow with foundation, then powder. For extra coverage, apply concealer before and after foundation. And try this eye-opening tip: Center a dot of shadow slightly lighter than the shade you've already used on your upper lid to subtly "open" the eye and distract attention from dark circles.

Your Skin Care Calendar

No matter what the season, here's the scoop on what you need to do to look your best.

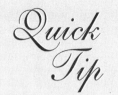

Quick Tip

A recent study has found that your skin's temperature increases while you sleep. That's good news if you want to deep moisturize or treat your skin. Because warmer skin absorbs more of the active ingredient of a product while you sleep, you get more bang for the buck at nighttime.

Quick Tip

If you are getting a glycolic acid peel in a dermatologist's office or a salon in the winter, watch out. You may be unable to tolerate as high a concentration of acid as you would in the summer. For example, you may tolerate 70 percent concentration of glycolic acid in August but no more than 40 percent in January. You may even opt to switch to the less irritating amino fruit acid peels. Ditto with your vitamin A topical products, such as Retin-A; you may need to switch to a less irritating form, such as Avita.

January

Right now, you are probably recovering from the holiday season (eating and drinking too much, not getting enough sleep) and its wear and tear on your skin. Make it your first New Year's resolution to take better care of your skin. Winter air can rob skin of its moisture, causing it to weaken and lose its capacity to repair itself. In fact, the skin is more sensitive in the winter, because it's drier and more dehydrated. So, your skin is probably crying out for more protection.

- Bump up your moisture levels by using milder (perhaps even creamier) cleansers and slightly richer moisturizers; those who aren't acne-prone can use slightly oil-based moisturizers.
- If you have sensitive skin or a condition such as eczema that gets worse in the winter, use a fragrance-free product (like Cetaphil lotion or cream).
- If you've been skiing or vacationing in the tropics, freshen up your complexion by exfoliating with home products or have a series of glycolic acid or amino fruit acid peels at a dermotologist's office.
- To keep your skin hydrated all over, apply a body moisturizer daily after bathing, while the skin is still damp. Glycolic acid moisturizers (like GlyDerm Body Lotion) help exfoliate skin and keep it smooth.
- Don't forget your hands; slather on a rich cream nightly and after every hand washing.
- If you've noticed a few bulges and are planning to undergo liposuction, now is the time to plan ahead to do it in February. (You don't want to end up wearing compression garments come July or August.)

February

Because the reflection of the sun's rays on the snow can be just as harmful (and wrinkle-causing) as a day on the beach, sunscreen is just as important in the winter, especially if you like skiing or other winter sports.

- Get in the habit of using at least an SPF 15 every day and a higher SPF if you'll be outdoors for more than 30 minutes.
- If you take a vacation to a warmer climate, make sure to wear an SPF 30, even if you're not on the beach.
- Please don't visit a tanning salon before you go; getting a "base tan" is just as damaging as lying in the sun.

- The other thing you may have noticed by now is unsightly spider veins and broken blood vessels on your nose. This is an ideal time to think about getting those zapped, so you'll be ready for spring.

March

- Keep up with your daily moisturizer and sunscreen!
- In anticipation of warm weather, accept the fact that sunbathing is taboo and learn how to apply self-tanner:

    1. Shower first and use an exfoliant on the rough skin of elbows and knees; otherwise, the tanner will show up darker on those areas of dead skin.
    2. After showering, pat skin completely dry with a soft towel.
    3. Slick a little petroleum jelly along hairline and over eyebrows to keep them from getting darkened from the tanner.
    4. Apply the tanner in smooth, long, and vertical, rather than horizontal, strokes to avoid streaking, blending well to avoid tell-tale marks.
    5. When you're done, wash your hands well to avoid tanning the palms of your hands!
    6. Let the tanner dry for about half an hour before you put on your clothes. You'll love your new glow.

April

Many women find that the change of seasons causes a flare of acne, partly due to warmer, less dry weather.

- Make the transition from cream to gel products; change to lighter, oil-free moisturizers.
- Add a glycolic acid product, if you haven't been using one; if all else fails, see your dermatologist.
- Don't pick at breakouts, as this can cause scarring.
- Large, painful cysts can be injected with a steroid to reduce inflammation.

May

- May is Skin Cancer Awareness Month. Schedule everyone in your family for an annual skin check, and let your dermatologist know about any moles or spots that are changing or a wound that won't heal.
- Learn to do a skin check on yourself; regular self-examination is the best way to become familiar with the many moles and spots on the skin.

Did you know that...

Sunscreen is a chemical agent that absorbs UV light to prevent sun rays from damaging the surrounding skin cells.

Sunblock is a chemical or physical agent that actually blocks the UV rays, causing them to bounce off the skin and reflect back. Zinc oxide, titanium dioxide, and specially designed SPF clothing are all examples of sun blocks.

Both these descriptions apply to UVA and UVB.

- With the help of a family member or friend, you should examine your skin, including hard-to-see areas such as your back. Inspect your moles and pay special attention to their sizes, shapes, edges, and color.
- A handy way to remember these features is to think of A, B, C, and D, which stand for Asymmetry, Border, Color, and Diameter. (See Chapter 6.)

June

Bathing suit season is here!

- If you were a little lazy about hair removal during the cold months, now is a good time to check out new hair removal methods, such as laser hair removal.
- Your feet will be on display more, so keep them looking neat by trimming nails and taking care of dead skin on the heels by using a pumice stone and then applying a rich moisturizer at least once a week.
- Don't ignore unattractive fungal infections under your toenails; a quick visit to your dermatologist can remove them pronto.
- And follow the sunscreen rule: apply it every day.

July

- Go through your medicine chest and throw out any sunscreens that are old. I recommend you purchase new sunscreen every year to ensure its effectiveness—some have a shelf life of only a year or two.
- Get your family, especially children, in the sunscreen habit, and stock up on waterproof sunblocks for your kids to take to camp.

August

- Learn to recognize poison ivy, oak, and sumac plants and stay away from them!
- A substance called urushiol, which is secreted from the leaves, causes a reaction wherever it touches your skin, and even a residue left on the handle of a gardening tool or on your pet can cause an infection days later.

September

- Many women want to begin treating unsightly varicose and spider veins on their legs in the spring, when they put on that first pair of shorts. However, the fall is a good time to undergo either sclerotherapy or laser treatment.

- To get the best results, we instruct our patients to wear waist-high, medical-grade compression stockings, which are much tighter than control pantyhose. The stockings are an important part of the treatment process, but can be unbearable to wear in the warmer months!
- If you live in a year-round warm climate, pick the season in which you'll be better able to tolerate the stockings for a week or so.

October

- If you haven't yet, consult with your dermatologist about in-office peels. These facial treatments are designed to smooth and refine the skin's texture, brighten a dull complexion, and help soften fine lines and wrinkles. Some acne patients find that regular treatments help control breakouts as well.
- Certain peels are even designed to eradicate pre-cancerous lesions that haven't yet appeared on the skin's surface. Glycolic acid, amino fruit acid, salicylic acid, microdermabrasion, and Jessner/Efudex treatments are all good for many skin types.
- Treatments administered in a doctor's office are different from those you will find at a spa, because they often utilize a higher concentration of active ingredient, may be offered only in a medical setting, and must be performed under medical supervision.

November

Get your skin glowing in time for the holidays!

- Review your skin-care routine by consulting with your doctor. Talk about what products you are using and how you are using them; whether they are giving you the results you are looking for, and whether anything new is available that you might benefit from.
- Don't use anyone else's prescription products, because they may cause an adverse effect.
- Visit a department store makeup counter and ask the cosmetician for some pointers on how to update your look.
- Get your makeup bag ready for the new year by discarding products that are past their prime. Ditch mascara after three months, eye pencils and foundation after a year.

December

You, hopefully, are keeping up with your exercise routine to maintain a healthy body and to fight off holiday weight gain!

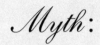

Myth:

You can "catch" poison ivy from someone else.

FACT:

You cannot "catch" or spread poison ivy, or poison sumac, or poison oak, from one person to another. A poison ivy skin breakout is an allergic reaction caused by a substance called urushiol, found in the sap of poison ivy, oak, and sumac. If you come into contact with urushiol, whether by touching the plant or a gardening tool, article of clothing, or even a pet that is carrying the sap, you may develop a reaction. Once the rash has developed on a person, that rash cannot be transmitted to another person. It is also a myth that "once allergic, always allergic." People who were particularly sensitive to poison ivy as children may not be allergic as adults.

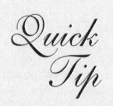

- If you work out in a gym, be aware that certain unwanted skin conditions can spread in a warm and moist environment like a locker room. Wear rubber sandals, instead of going barefoot, to avoid exposure to a wart virus, and wipe off equipment before and after you use it for general skin hygiene.
- If you prefer working out outdoors, protect your face and skin to prevent chapping and broken blood vessels.

Cold Weather Rules

Realize that when it's cold, there is simply less moisture in the air. The air seeks moisture, pulling it out from every place–including your skin. As a result you get flaky, scaly skin and a pale, dull complexion.

- Always keep in mind that you need to protect and soothe your skin, which has been buffeted about by the elements.
- To avoid getting cracked dry spots on your skin, apply moisturizer in layers. First apply one layer; after letting it dry, apply another on top of it.
- Avoid using products with alcohol.
- Switch to cleansing with nondrying gentle cleansers and use a moisturizing mask once a week.
- Use a heavier, non-water-based sunscreen.
- Try a glycolic acid product to lock in moisture.
- Get a good lip balm to protect the delicate skin on your lips.
- To avoid broken blood vessels on your face from sudden changes in temperature, wrap a scarf around your face when you're outdoors. It will also help protect you against windburn.
- Often your skin can look paler in the winter. Switch your foundation to a lighter, more appropriate color, or go the other way and get color from a tube of self-tanner.

Warm Weather Rules

In the summer, breakouts can occur when pores get clogged and when sebum and debris react with bacteria. Air conditioning can also rob your skin of moisture because the system pulls moisture from the air, which then dehydrates your skin.

- In the summer, your skin is better hydrated because of the humidity.
- Your skin is hardier during these times (because it is better hydrated) and will tolerate a heavier concentration of products than in the winter.
- If you are oily and acne-prone, you may want to start using benzyol peroxide products (which can be too drying in the winter). Just do

the patch test (see Chapter 4) to make sure you are not allergic (1 percent to 5 percent of the population is allergic to benzoyl peroxide).
- Switch from cream products to gel products. Why? A cream is more emollient and moisturizing, and a gel can be slightly more drying.

Makes Good Skin Sense No Matter the Season

- Wear a sunscreen to protect against harmful UV rays, which can be intensified by the reflections from snow and ice.
- Hot showers can irritate sensitive, delicate skin. Reduce the time you spend in the shower and lower the temperature.
- Wear sunglasses when outdoors to keep you from getting wrinkles from squinting into the sun.
- Dry heat indoors can zap skin of needed moisture. Fight back with a humidifier.
- After working out, ditch your usual session in the sauna.

Did you know that…

Why do you feel so good in the sun? A study at Boston University shows that sunlight makes your skin produce beta-endorphins, the chemicals that create a natural high. What has yet to be determined is how much exposure you need to produce this effect.

chapter four

Complexion Perfection

The most beautiful thing we can experience is the mysterious.
—ALBERT EINSTEIN

HEALTHY, GLOWING SKIN IS EASILY ONE OF THE BEST BEAUTY ASSETS A WOMAN CAN have. Ideally, you want your skin to look great all year round, not just during the summer, winter, or on special occasions. That's why it's essential to nip in the bud skin care problems that might crop up. In this chapter, I'll cover the major skin care problems—such as teen acne, adult acne, hormonal acne, or other "acne imitators"—explain why they develop, and provide you with easy, sound solutions for getting-rid of them. You'll also learn the best way to zap a zit—any time, and how to beat the most destructive beauty burglars—the sun, lack of sleep, smoking, drinking, and stress. I'll even give you an easy key for figuring out your skin's real age—not just the age you think you see when you look in the mirror. With this information, you'll be able to face with confidence any skin care problems that arise.

Causes of Acne

To best understand why acne happens, picture this: Most of our skin is covered with tiny follicles that contain oil-producing sebaceous glands. Along with these sebaceous glands, we also have tiny hairs growing up inside small canals within each follicle. The place on the skin's surface where each follicular canal opens is called a pore.

Clear skin (without eruptions) occurs when the cells lining the canal shed regularly and are carried out by the oil produced by the sebaceous glands through the pore to the skin's surface. A problem begins when cells clump together, causing a plug. Then the excess oil being produced by the sebaceous glands starts to build up behind the plug. At the same time, the normal bacteria in the follicle start to

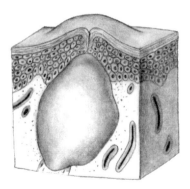

NODULAR ACNE

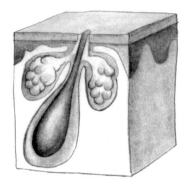

NORMAL HAIR FOLLICLE

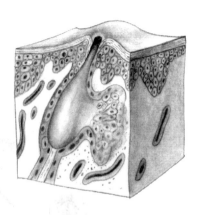

BLACKHEAD

increase, feeding on the oil and blocking the pore. When the blockage, or plug, reaches the surface of the skin, it appears as a blackhead, caused when the dead skin cells and oil fill the pore and are visible. Plugs that remain just below the skin's surface are whiteheads.

Many people have inflammatory acne, which occurs when the skin bacteria produce irritating substances that may break into the skin surrounding the follicle. Then, "pus pimples" (small pus-filled lumps), papules (small red lumps that protrude above the skin's surface), nodules (large red lumps that protrude above the skin's surface), and cysts may form. This type of acne, called cystic acne, is the most severe and requires treatment by a dermatologist.

Fluctuating hormones can also contribute to acne breakouts, which is why teenagers tend to break out, why women break out around their periods, and why women may break out during pregnancy and postpartum. Hormones cause oil glands to enlarge and to produce more oil during puberty and throughout the teen years. Also, during those years, the follicle wall thickens and cells clump together, blocking the follicular canal. The areas with the largest, most active oil glands–the forehead, nose, and chin (T-zone)–are most likely to develop acne. But acne can also develop on the neck, back, shoulders, and chest.

In addition, anything that puts pressure on certain parts of the skin may bring on what's called "friction acne." This term applies to blemishes that occur where pressure is applied to skin, such as around the mouth of a flute player or on the side of the face and around the chin of people who spend considerable time on the phone, cradling it with their face and chin.

Teen Acne

This type of acne normally shows up in teenagers between the ages of 10 and 20. It is characterized by blackheads, whiteheads, papules, pustules, cysts, and nodules that erupt on the face in the T-zone and on the inner cheeks (nearest the nose). This type of acne occurs because of the hormonal changes that take place during puberty.

Adult Acne

There are two sub-types of adult acne. The first looks like teen acne, but it occurs in women and men over the age of 20. The second type, hormonal acne, is caused by fluctuating hormones and consists of cysts and nodules that frequently don't come to a head. Hormonal acne is distributed more along the jawline, chin, and upper and outer neck area.

Acne-Troubled Skin

If you suffer from acne, don't despair. There are many, many ways to treat the condition. Some of the most common methods include using topical preparations or oral, or systemic, agents. For topical treatments, you can find a number of effective agents available over the counter and many with a prescription. One of the most popular topical treatments, which has been around for decades, is benzoyl peroxide. It's a terrific ingredient for several reasons: You can get it without a prescription; most pharmacies carry it; and it is the active agent in many pricey acne products that are sold in department stores and over the Internet. Other topical acne treatments include salicylic acid, vitamin A, and, of course, alpha hydroxy acids. If I had to pick one for the first choice, it would be benzoyl peroxide, because it's the only one that is antibacterial and also exfoliates skin, unblocks pores, and dries up excess oil.

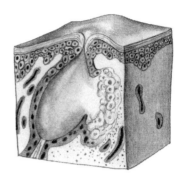

WHITEHEAD

Are You Allergic?

There are only two drawbacks to using benzoyl peroxide products. One, they can be slightly drying and irritating, so it's a good idea to choose a strength that's not too irritating for the skin; if you're not sure, stick with a 5 percent concentration. The other drawback is a big, though rare, one. Approximately 5 percent of the population is allergic to benzoyl peroxide and will react to the product by breaking out in an itchy, scaly rash, resembling the one you get from poison ivy.

Other Choices

If you find you are allergic to benzoyl peroxide, you may choose to use one of a few other over-the-counter anti-acne agents, including glycolic acid and the rest of the alpha hydroxy acid family. These agents work by exfoliating the skin, opening up the pores, and allowing the sebum from the sebaceous glands to come up freely to the skin's surface, where it can get cleansed off, rather than allowing it to hang around and block the pores. Another very effective acid, which comes in a wide variety of cleansers, creams, and masks, and works well at exfoliating skin and unblocking clogged pores, is a beta hydroxy acid called salicylic acid.

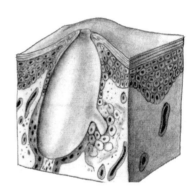

PUSTULE

Many women swear by another over-the-counter agent, retinol, to help their acne. Like tretinoin in Retin-A (see Chapter 11), retinol is from the vitamin A family and can help increase exfoliation and normalize the cells that line the pores so they don't get blocked down below the surface. When you have acne, the cells lining the pores clump together and form a plug that blocks the pores below the surface of the skin. Vitamin A gets down there and normalizes this abnormality so that the cells do what mother nature intended, which is to come up through the pores and out onto the skin's surface along with the sebum.

Program for Acne-Troubled Skin

To treat your condition:

- Wash your skin with a cleanser containing salicylic acid (such as SalAc Wash, Neutrogena Oil-Free Acne Wash, or Oil of Olay Age Defying Series Daily Renewal Cleanser).
- Apply an oil-free moisturizer with an SPF 15 or higher. Choose products that contain glycolic acid or another alpha hydroxy acid. This gives a double benefit: the alpha hydroxy acid opens pores as it sloughs off dead skin cells, while it simultaneously moisturizes the skin. Oil-free moisturizers that have SPF 15 and also contain alpha hydroxy acids include NeoStrata, Neutrogena, and Purpose.
- In the evening, cleanse with a cleanser containing alpha hydroxy and apply a cream containing benzoyl peroxide (such as Oxy5, Clearasil, or Neutrogena On-the-Spot Acne Treatment).

Guerrilla Tactics to Fight Acne

- Clean your face at least twice a day, especially if you perspire heavily. Use a mild cleanser for in between cleansing, such as after working out.
- Use only makeup and moisturizers that are noncomedogenic and use only oil-free sunscreens.
- Clean your cosmetic brushes and makeup pads with soapy water at least two or three times a week.
- Avoid touching your face during the day. Keep in mind that hands are full of microscopic bacteria that can transfer to your face and aggravate your condition. Also, wash your hands after handling money, which has been shown to contain a great amount of bacteria and germs.
- Remove all your makeup before going to bed.
- Change your pillowcases at least every few days and wash your sheets often.
- Avoid resting your face on the telephone, a good breeder for bacteria.
- Cleanse your telephone with an alcohol pad.

How Do I Know I Have Adult Acne?

Adult acne is becoming a huge problem with women (and some men) over the age of 20. A surprisingly large number of patients suffering from adult acne, the majority of them women, come into my office complaining of acne breakouts for the first time. Others with the problem see it as a continuation of their "teenage acne phase." Regardless of whether the breakouts are recurrent or new, they can make you feel horrible about the way you look and wreak havoc on your self-esteem and social life.

Did you know that...

Contrary to popular belief, sunbathing makes zits worse, not better. The initial, temporary drying effect—and the blemish-concealing tan—may fool you, but UV rays actually stimulate oil production. At the same time, they thicken the outer layer of your skin, which blocks your pores and leads to breakouts.

When patients say they have adult acne, I first check to make certain that what they think they have is the correct diagnosis. Many conditions can imitate or mimic adult acne, such as rosacea (see Chapter 1), yeast infections of the hair follicles, and breakouts resulting from pores that have been blocked by oil-based makeup products or leave-in hair products, such as hairspray, mousse, and gel.

In women, the facial lesions may be present all the time or may flare up only in the week directly preceding the start of the menstrual cycle. Why is the week before the menstrual cycle crucial? That is the time during which the progesterone spike occurs. Progesterone is the female hormone that induces ovulation, and it closely resembles the male hormone testosterone. Because the hormone is similar in its chemical makeup to testosterone, it works the same way in stimulating the oil glands, resulting in acne flare-ups prior to ovulation.

Prescription Topical Products to Fight Acne

- If you are looking for a prescription topical solution, you can ask your doctor to prescribe one of several remedies, including topical antibiotics, such as clindamycin or erythromycin. These antibiotics work to fight the bacteria that form pimples after the pore has gotten blocked.
- If you aren't allergic to sulfur, some sulfur-containing products can work very effectively by causing mild drying, exfoliating the skin, and acting as an antibacterial agent.
- If you want to go to a stronger, more effective vitamin A product than over-the-counter retinol, you may decide to choose a treatment from the prescription-strength vitamin A products, such as Retin-A, Avita, Differin, and Tazorac.

Azelex is another topical prescription product which has antibacterial, anti-inflammatory, and exfoliating properties. It contains 20 percent azelaic acid, a natural substance derived from wheat and grain. What's great about Azelex is that it also has the ability to correct pigmentation problems, such as melasma and freckles. It doesn't work like a bleaching agent (which lightens everything it touches, including normal skin), but instead goes into the areas where you are heavily pigmented and tones it down without affecting the rest of the skin. It also helps to rid the skin of the redness caused by acne. People with darker complexions can use it to correct any pigmentation changes that happen after a pimple has healed and left a dark brown spot that can last for months. Azelex attacks all problems at once, plus it helps protect you from getting pimples in the first place.

Quick Tip

To test if you are allergic to benzoyl peroxide, take a tiny amount and apply it to the skin of your inner forearm, just below the elbow crease. The skin there is just as sensitive as the skin on your face. Do this every evening for two or three nights in a row. If your skin becomes red and itchy, it's a sure sign you are allergic, so don't put the benzoyl peroxide on your face.

Quick Tip

Rule of thumb to follow: If you have acne, ease up on the salt. High iodine intake can result in acne on the face, chest, and back.

Prescription Oral Products to Fight Acne

There are a number of oral agents available that treat adult acne and these can be divided into several categories.

Oral Antibiotics

The oldest of the oral acne medications is tetracycline. It has two derivatives, doxycycline and minocycline, which also help to kill the bacteria that cause acne. Because it's possible for patients to develop bacterial resistance to antibiotics, I prefer to use these oral agents only for a short period of time. Antibiotics kill the bacteria in acne, and are also anti-inflammatory. Other oral antibiotics used include erythromycin, Bactrim, amoxicillin, and Zithromax.

Hormone Therapy

If your adult acne flares up in response to your menstrual cycle, then hormone therapy can be extremely helpful. Hormone therapy is available in two forms: birth-control pills and a hormone-blocking agent called Aldactone.

I recommend taking a course of birth-control pills to help control hormonally driven acne. Birth-control pills work by suppressing the patient's own hormones and substituting them with synthetic derivatives, which don't stimulate the oil glands and acne flare-ups.

A dermatologist can predict how to treat a patient who has hormonal acne by listening to her history. For example, if someone tells me that her acne is the same 30 days out of the month, I would tend to direct her to a course of treatment of Accutane, rather than to a hormone treatment. On the other hand, if a woman tells me her skin is completely clear three weeks out of the month, with flare-ups occurring only the week before her period, I would recommend she take either Ortho Tri-Cyclen birth-control pills or Aldactone. Many patients overlap both groups, suffering from acne all of the time, with additional flare-ups around their menstrual cycle. For these patients, I basically customize a routine to address both the problems of circulating hormones as well as the blocking up of their sebaceous oil glands.

Birth-control pills, specifically Ortho Tri-Cyclen, have been approved by the FDA not only to help prevent pregnancy, but also to help control adult acne. Other birth-control pills that have been shown to be effective at regulating hormonal acne include Ortho-Cept, Desogen, Demulen, and Ortho-Cyclen, among others.

For women who are experiencing definite hormonal flares but don't wish to take birth-control pills, Aldactone often works effectively to balance hormones. Aldactone is not itself a hormone; rather, it blocks the hormone receptor on the sebaceous oil gland so that the receptor doesn't recognize the woman's own hormones.

The Accutane Equation

The ultimate medication for adult acne, as well as teenage acne, is Accutane, which is, in my opinion, one of the greatest drugs that has ever been invented. Unfortunately, Accutane has been much maligned in its recent history. It was approved in 1982 by the FDA, so it has been available in this country for 20 years. The standard therapy for either adult acne or teenage acne is a five-month course of two pills of Accutane a day. Most people report that taking a course of treatment of Accutane results in a dramatic clearing of their acne and that it's very unusual for the acne to come back.

What's the Problem? The reason people are wary of Accutane, and it's a very real reason, is that it has been proven to be a potent teratogen (causer of birth defects). However, there is a misunderstanding implicit in that statement that has led to widespread rumors and myths about the drug. It is very clearly known at this point that the risk of Accutane-related birth defects exists only if a woman is taking the medication while she is pregnant. The key point here is: the woman needs to be pregnant and taking the drug at the same time. Accutane is rapidly eliminated from a person's system. Therefore, if a woman waits one month and one menstrual cycle after completing a course of Accutane treatment before conceiving, the medication will be completely out of her system and won't affect any future pregnancy. Because Accutane is a member of the vitamin A family, it affects how cells differentiate and divide, which means that it can affect only a developing fetus. It is important to know that Accutane has no effect, whatsoever, on a man's sperm or a woman's eggs.

Possible Side Effects. Patients can experience a few other side effects of taking Accutane, depending on the dose. These potential effects include dry lips, dry skin, slight sun sensitivity, and slight stiffness of the muscles and joints when exercising intensely. Still, in my experience of treating more than three thousand patients with Accutane, none of these reactions has ever led any patient to discontinue Accutane therapy.

Big Benefits. Another benefit of Accutane is that the course regimens can be customized to meet patients' needs. For example, some adult patients, especially women, will complete a five-month course of treatment and end up with a few mild acne breakouts. For these patients, I've tried other regimens, which have worked well, including very, very, low doses of Accutane daily for one to three months, followed by an off-Accutane rest period, followed by one to three months of Accutane, and so on, on and off. Other times, I'll prescribe another type of low-dose Accutane routine, which can consist of the patient taking just one pill per week.

Quick Tip

If you have acne, make sure to wash your facecloth often. Otherwise, you are simply wiping oil, dirt, grime, and makeup on freshly washed skin, creating a breeding ground for pimples and acne.

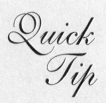

Accutane and Chemical Peeling. I've found that very low-dose Accutane can actually enhance the results of mild chemical peeling or microdermabrasion, contrary to some standard warnings. The warnings say that patients on Accutane are at an increased risk of scarring, because of Accutane's effect on the sebaceous oil gland, where the new cells come from. I've found that if I use a low-dose Accutane of 10 milligrams a day combined with a light glycolic-acid or fruit-acid peel and/or microdermabrasion, the results are wonderful, because of the "thinned down" effect of the outer skin-cell layer. So, I occasionally recommend combining Accutane with peeling or microdermabrasion, as long as you are under the care of a skilled doctor who is experienced in Accutane as well as in chemical peeling.

The Appeal of Glycolic Facials

Some practitioners promote other ways to treat acne, which I don't necessarily agree with. Many suggest mild facials or glycolic acid treatments to exfoliate acne-ridden skin, but I think you should instead select one of the many effective medications available to address the problem. Personally, I also feel that glycolic facial treatments or other facials are far too time- and cost-intensive as the primary part of acne therapy. They have no long-term anti-acne benefits, because four weeks after your last facial treatment, your pores will begin to block up again.

These facials can provide wonderful treatments for the complexion, and they can help considerably with sun damage and in reducing fine wrinkles, but I don't recommend them as a priority treatment for acne. I do make one exception to this rule: pregnant or nursing women, who are limited in terms of choosing preparations that are safe while pregnant or nursing. In these special, very limited, situations, I usually suggest the patient try treating her adult acne with mild topical solutions and glycolic acid or other exfoliating facial treatments. But these limited situations are the only ones for which I'd recommend glycolic peels as part of a regular acne routine.

Acne Imitators

Another condition that causes breakouts is called perioral (around the mouth area) acne. This noncontagious condition occurs primarily in women aged 25 to 45 years, and can usually be recognized by pimply/rashy eruptions that crop up on the chin, around the mouth, the lower part of the nose, and under and around the eyes. It is caused by overgrowth of bacteria that normally live on the skin, minding their own business. Perioral acne breakouts often appear after the woman is stressed, has had sun exposure, or has been using too heavy or occlusive makeup or moisturizing products. A breakout can even come after a cold, flu, or other illness. Often misdiagnosed as an inflammation, these breakouts are often subsequently treated with cortisone type creams—which just make the condition worse, even though such treatment may make the skin feel better temporarily.

How to Treat Perioral Acne

- Stop putting on cortisone creams and moisturizer.
- Keep your hands away from your face.
- Gently wash your face with a mild antibacterial cleanser.
- Try to limit the amount of stress in your life.
- If the condition persists after a few days, you need a dermatologist to prescribe a topical (or oral) antibiotic.

Is It Your Hairspray?

Sometimes hormonal acne looks like something else that I call "hairspray acne." This type of breakout occurs when leave-in hair-styling products, such as sprays, mousses, and gels, flake off onto the sides of the face and neck during the day. This "migration" can end up blocking the pores in these areas and lead to acne and ugly cysts. I always say when a woman comes to see me who has mostly cysts and nodules along her jawline and side of her neck, it's H or H acne—hairspray or hormones.

Basically, if your acne flares up or gets worse with your menstrual cycle, there is a hormonal component to it. If you don't think it's hormonally based (meaning it doesn't flare up around your cycle), but it looks the way I described hormonal acne as looking, then you may want to avoid using leave-in hair products, including two-in-one shampoo/conditioner products, which are responsible for breakouts in many people.

Yeast Acne

Your skin can also break out from a superficial yeast infection of the hair follicles. In fact, a yeast fungus called pityrosporum lives in your hair follicles' sebaceous oil glands, where it usually resides in such small numbers that it causes no problem. Occasionally, the yeast overgrows and causes dandruff (seborrhea), redness, itching, and/or dryness of the scalp—as well as an eruption of red bumps and pus pimples on your face that look like acne, but are caused by the yeast.

A good way to figure out whether you have a yeast infection of the hair follicles is to notice where you break out. Yeast infections tend to occur more often on the forehead, jawline, neck, and along the hairline, rather than on the mid-face. Some people also break out in pimples on the nape of the neck area and in places where long hair can touch, such as sideburns and shoulders.

To fix it, try Nizoral shampoo (which is anti-yeast) over the counter, shampoo a few times a week, and while in the shower, let it stream over your face, directly onto the affected areas. If the eruption goes away in a couple of weeks, it was caused by yeast; if not, it's probably acne.

A Reason to Help

According to a study funded by Neutrogena, 46 percent of teenagers with mild to moderate facial acne reported that acne had a damaging effect on their physical self-image. Twenty-seven percent said it had negatively impacted their social life.

Acne-Prone Shopping Cart Checklist
Avoid these ingredients and products, which can make you break out:

Any oils, especially mineral oil, safflower oil, peanut oil
Petrolatum
Lanolin
Artificial fragrance and colors
S.D. alcohol

- To help a pimple heal faster, soothe the skin with a cool compress.
- To hide a pimple, dab on a sheer water-based concealer or oil-free foundation. Follow with another tiny dab of concealer and then dust the area with loose, translucent powder for a no-shine finish.

A Reason to Glow

Based on new research, cited in the book *The Survival of the Prettiest* by Dr. Nancy Etcoff, a psychologist at Massachusetts General Hospital and a teacher at Harvard Medical School, men have historically viewed women whose skin wasn't smooth and glowing (read, had acne, wrinkles, or sun-damaged skin) with caution. That's because, in prehistoric times women who had breakouts and whose skin wasn't smooth and glowing were often carriers of parasites—obviously, not a man's first choice for the mother of his future children. Scientists say this prehistoric instinct is carried in our genes, which explains why beauty is not just the product of what society (and magazines) tell us it is. Measures of beauty are, in fact, also intrinsic to human nature.

How to Zap a Zit

Here's my professional opinion on the best way to zap a zit: Find a way to prevent it from forming in the first place! What many people don't realize is that it can take as long as eight weeks from the time a pore gets blocked to the time it erupts on the skin in the form of a pimple. In effect, by the time you are painstakingly applying topical products to a pimple that has broken out on your skin, it's about eight weeks too late. That's why, if you are at all prone to breakouts, it's a good idea to put together a daily routine designed to prevent breakouts in the first place. But if you can't wait, have a major date or presentation, and need quick relief, pick up some 10 percent benzoyl peroxide (as long as you're not one of the 5 percent of the population who is allergic to it). No other product can beat the potent drying, exfoliating, and antibacterial effects of 10 percent benzoyl peroxide (found in Clearasil and Oxy-10). Save your money and avoid buying any product, especially an expensive "designer" or "brand name" product, that has less than 10 percent of this active ingredient. All you need to zap a zit very quickly is a tiny dot of 10 percent benzoyl peroxide, two to three times a day.

If your zit is more like a cyst (a slightly deeper lesion), then you may also want to try applying warm compresses. Simply wet a washcloth, handkerchief, or any clean, soft cloth with warm water and gently hold it to the cyst or pimple for several minutes at a time, several times a day. If worse comes to worst, and your pimple or cyst is especially large, or if you have a hot date, important party, big presentation, or even wedding pictures and can't spare the time to wait a day or two for the pimple to heal and disappear, then I recommend you make a quick trip to the dermatologist for a little cortisone injection. This will usually zap the zit or cyst within 24 hours.

The Right Way to Squeeze

While dermatologists always caution against the evils of squeezing zits (*you'll make them worse; you'll scar; it doesn't help*), the truth is, people do squeeze their pimples. They can't help themselves. I think part of it is the social anxiety caused by having an unsightly eruption marring your facial beauty and part of it is that people have an urge to self-treat, hoping the zit will just pop and go away.

I'm here to tell you it's possible, but only—and I repeat *only*—if you pop your pimple in the most hygienic way possible. Here's what you need to do: Go to your local pharmacy and for a few bucks ($5 to $15), pick up something called a comedone extractor (translation, pimple popper or zit zapper). These are usually small, metal devices with a small cup on one end and a hole in the bottom. To use the comedone extractor, first disinfect both the pimple and the extractor by cleaning them with rubbing alcohol. Then gently place the zit zapper over the pus pimple and press down firmly. This will usually open up the pimple and discharge the pus without scarring or driving the infection deeper into the skin. This way is far better than squeezing your pimple between two fingers, which can actually cause infection by driving the pus from the pimple into deeper tissues.

The Truth about Tea Tree Oil

Many people rush out to buy products containing tea tree oil to treat their breakouts. Here's what I think: Though tea tree oil works as an anti-

Quick Tip

Zap a zit fast by combining one-quarter teaspoon of table salt with one cup of lukewarm water. Dip a piece of gauze or tissue into the mixture, then lightly press it against the blemish for one minute. The salt solution will bring down swelling and lessen redness. To speed healing, follow with an over-the-counter treatment product containing 10 percent of benzoyl peroxide or salicylic acid.

inflammatory and is also antibacterial, it has a serious flaw when it comes to treating breakouts–the oil itself may block pores. Still, if you've used tea tree oil successfully in the past to zap your zits and find it hasn't blocked your pores, then by all means continue to do what works for you. I don't recommend it as an acne therapy to my patients, because I feel many other superior products are already available for them to choose from.

Beat the Beauty Burglars

Many other things can contribute to a less than ideal complexion, besides pimples and blemishes.

First, a pop quiz: What's the number one thing that will rob the skin of its beauty, make it look rough and blotchy, and cause you to look years older than you are? If you haven't figured it out by now, it's the sun. I'm sure I sound like a broken record, but I must repeat myself, because it's so important for you to take in this information.

The sun ages the skin rapidly, powerfully, cumulatively, and indiscriminately. Because it directly affects multiple skin layers, the sun can cause splotchy coloring and broken blood vessels. Over time, cumulative sun exposure can damage the collagen (the springy support structure of the skin), causing sagging and wrinkles. Skin that has been spared the damage of sun exposure simply looks better, healthier, and definitely younger.

So, how do you handle this sneaky beauty burglar? Sunscreen, sunscreen, and more sunscreen. Apply an SPF of at least 15 daily. Find one that protects against both ultraviolet UVA and UVB rays. And ignore the myths that "It doesn't wash off," "It's waterproof," and the ever popular, "Well, I already had some sun, so why bother now?" (For more on sun, see Chapter 12.)

Smoking is the next big beauty burglar. We know that smoking is bad for our skin, but what exactly does it do to it and how? Smoking affects the distribution of oxygen in the blood to skin cells in the same way it affects the heart's circulation–by preventing the cells from getting the oxygen and nutrients they need. Because it allows less oxygen to get to the skin's cells, smokers (as well as those who inhale lots of secondhand smoke, as at a nightclub) often look pasty-faced. If you smoke, you are undermining even the best attempts to maintain a youthful, healthy complexion. You also are likely to get unattractive smoker's lines around your mouth. Another negative effect of smoking is that it markedly lengthens the time it takes for a wound to heal, which you need to consider if you are considering any kind of facial surgery or other rejuvenating procedure.

Stress is the third beauty burglar. When you are stressed, your blood vessels constrict, causing increased wear and tear on the cardiovascular system.

Stress also makes you release all sorts of stress hormones, which, in the ancient fight-or-flight response, also trigger your body to decide that skin circulation is not a priority and to channel blood away from the skin toward muscles and other organs of the body. This stress response worked well enough for our ancestors who were avoiding being a meal ticket for predators, but it can wreak havoc on our bodies today. If you chronically stress yourself out, you not only make yourself, and everybody else around you, nuts, but you also deprive your skin of crucial oxygen and nutrients and aggravate any skin condition you may already have, such as eczema or acne.

Lack of sleep is the fourth beauty burglar. Sleep is absolutely essential to looking your best. If you don't get your 40 winks, you'll pay for it with a droopy-looking face. Why? As your systems try to shut down, muscles become fatigued, and the face begins to sag and droop. Your skin can also take on a sallow appearance, as your pulse and blood pressure drop, causing less blood to pump into the face—not an attractive way to look.

Poor diet is yet another beauty burglar (see Chapter 8). Basically, if you don't eat a well-balanced diet and don't provide your body with the correct vitamins and nutrients, your skin won't look its best. You also need to drink lots of water (eight 8-ounce glasses per day). Not drinking enough water causes your skin to become dry and flaky. Here's how to tell if you are getting enough: Slowly increase your water intake until you notice you're making more frequent trips to the ladies' room. Our kidneys regulate our bodies' water balance. Once we have more water than we need, our kidneys excrete the excess.

Alcohol (and not the rubbing kind) is the final beauty burglar. Drinking too much alcohol (the difference between one cocktail and six beers) does a number on the skin. First, the blood vessels dilate, which creates more broken blood vessels (a reason drinkers often have red, bloodshot eyes). Second, drinking too much can make you retain water, because the blood vessels become so dilated, the heart pumps more fluid into the surrounding tissues. This makes you feel and look bloated. Not a pretty picture.

Beating Back the Beauty Burglars

Beating back the beauty burglars is a matter of making the right lifestyle decisions. Limit your sun exposure and use sunscreen. Don't start smoking and stop if you already do. Try to control the amount of stress in your life or learn coping mechanisms for reducing stress. Get plenty of rest, eat a healthy, balanced diet, and drink alcholic beverages in moderation.

If you follow this advice, you'll look better longer than most of the people you know, who don't do a thing to fight the beauty burglars before they rob them of their youth, beauty, and, ultimately, their good health.

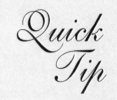

Quick Tip

A good rule of thumb when shopping for an over-the-counter anti-acne or complexion-clearing product is to check whether the active ingredient is benzoyl peroxide in a 5 or 10 percent concentration.

Myth:

You can get acne from your diet, your sex life (or lack of one), or dirt.

FACT:

Acne is not caused by diet, sex (or the lack thereof), or dirt. Acne can be caused or aggravated by menstruation and/or pregnancy (due to changes in hormone levels), sweating, humidity, some medications, and certain cosmetics or hair preparations.

Determining Your Skin's Real Age

Most Americans get it wrong when they interpret the brown spots, color changes, fine lines, wrinkles, and broken capillaries they see when they look in the mirror as signs of aging. In fact, all of these skin problems are signs of sun damage or photo aging, which has nothing to do with true aging. Chronological aging often reflects gravity changes, muscle changes, and to some extent, the movement or loss of support of filler tissue, which causes skin to sag. Everything else is caused by the sun.

To figure out how much sun damage you have, just look at your outer arm, the part that lines up with the back of your hand. This is considered to be a primary sun-exposed area. Now, slowly rotate your arm from a palm-down position outward, until your palm faces up and your thumb points out, away from you. With your other hand, lift up the upper inner arm skin, just below the armpit. Take a good look at that patch of skin and compare the difference between the skin in that area (which has been virtually protected from the sun most of your life) and the area on your outer arm. If the two look virtually the same, in terms of color, freckles, and texture, then you've probably had very little sun damage or photo aging, and your appearance is true to your chronological age. If, however, like most of us, you see a distinct difference between the soft, smooth skin of the upper inner arm and the upper-outer arm (which is browner, less glowing, more freckly, more leathery), then you can assess how much sun damage you actually have. Also, if both your inner and outer arms and your face look about the same, then the facial changes are most likely related to aging.

The Color in Your Skin

If your skin has changed color recently, it is a warning sign that you need to pay attention to what's going on.

If your skin is red: It means your skin is inflamed and irritated. For example, sunburn will cause your skin to flush red. Redness in the center of the face (cheeks, nose, and chin) accompanied by pimples may indicate rosacea, a skin disease involving blood vessels. Spicy foods, caffeine, alcohol, stress, heat, and certain birth-control pills can aggravate rosacea. Antibiotics or blood pressure medications (like Clonidine or Corgard) may be taken for a few months to stabilize the condition, after which it might disappear for up to two years. Chronic redness without pimples and across the nose and cheeks in a butterfly shape may signal lupus erythematosus, an autoimmune disease that requires medical attention. In that case, see your doctor.

If your skin is sallow: It could mean you haven't been sleeping enough, in which case the cure is apparent—get some shut-eye. Sun damage could also be the cause, as could smoking, which reduces blood supply, causing the skin to look sallow. Brighten your complexion with a cream or lotion containing retinol or alpha hydroxy acid (AHA) or with a vitamin C serum.

If your skin pales: This happens when the skin's pigment cells are destroyed or damaged in some way, causing the body to produce less pigment. For example, skin often looks lighter after a rash, sunburn, heat burn, or sore. This is called postinflammatory hypopigmentation, a loss of pigmentation due to inflammation. It's most common in darker complexions. Exfoliating may make it worse. The best way to approach this problem is to use sun protection on the damaged areas and on the surrounding skin. (The unaffected skin will likely darken faster in response to sunlight than will the affected lighter areas, making the difference between them even more noticeable.) You can also use alpha hydroxy or vitamin A compounds to help normalize the differences in pigmentation. If the affected area continues to increase, you may have vitiligo, an autoimmune disease, and should see a doctor.

The 10 Commandments of Skin Care
Follow these rules, and you'll keep time on your side.

1. Wear a sunscreen that protects against both UVA and UVB rays every day. The main cause of skin aging and wrinkles is incidental exposure to the sun (when you're driving, walking, etc.).
2. Don't smoke. Smoking causes the skin to age prematurely and saps the skin of oxygen. It also causes the skin to look sallow and unattractive (due to the lack of oxygen).
3. Avoid drinking alcohol. Like smoking, drinking too much alcohol dehydrates the skin and can cause the skin to age prematurely.
4. Keep stress down to a minimum. Excess stress can contribute to premature aging by preventing nutrients and oxygen from reaching your skin.
5. Drink lots of water, about eight 8-ounce glasses a day.
6. Get enough sleep. Our body repairs and rejuvenates itself while we sleep.
7. Eat a healthy, well-balanced diet.
8. Move your body. Regular exercise increases the flow of nutrients and oxygen to the skin, giving it a healthy glow.
9. Wear sunglasses. This will protect the eyes and the delicate skin around them. Check the label to make sure the lenses provides UVA and UVB protection.
10. Take short showers and baths in warm rather than hot water, to avoid further dehydrating and irritating the skin.

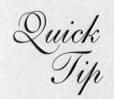

Quick Tip

If you think you have a sensitivity to any of your cosmetics products (your skin breaks out, gets irritated and rashy), you may have contaminated the product by touching it with your fingers. A better bet is to find applicators and bottles that allow you to squeeze or pour the products onto the tip of the finger, rather than reaching into the bottle.

chapter five

The Question Corner

I'm attracted to obstacles I need to overcome.
—MADONNA

THIS CHAPTER IS DEVOTED TO ANSWERING YOUR MOST COMMON SKIN CARE, BEAUTY, and medical questions.

Q: Is it true that daily facial exercises will prevent wrinkling?

A: Facial wrinkles occur due to two factors: gravity pulling on muscles and the natural breakdown of skin elasticity due to aging. (Lack of moisture and sun exposure accelerate the effects of gravity and aging.) Facial exercises pull skin too much, and once skin begins to lose elasticity, wrinkles can develop. Constantly furrowing the brow, squinting, or puckering your lips—even smiling—will create wrinkles or worsen those you have. Can wrinkles be erased? Yes, with Retin-A, alpha hydroxy acids, chemical peels, Botox, laser resurfacing, plastic surgery, dermabrasion, and filler injections, such as collagen, fat, Dermologen, and Gortex. Repetitive facial exercises can actually aggravate, rather than prevent, wrinkles.

Q: How do I fix my sun-damaged skin?

A: Over time, the sun erodes the skin's ability to produce collagen, slowing it down until the skin loses its elasticity. Sun damage is basically cumulative, which means that 70 percent of it comes from casual exposure, such as from walking down the street, driving a car, and riding a bike. Every tiny little bit of exposure adds up in your sun bank, until voilà, you reach the point that the bank is full, and your skin suffers sun damage.

First of all, to nip the ongoing problem in the bud and to reduce future damage, look for sunscreens that give you both UVA and UVB protection. Glycolic acid peels are mild, but can create a subtle improvement in the skin by sloughing off damaged skin cells.

Also get a prescription for a vitamin A derivative topical, such as Retin-A, which helps get rid of wrinkles and reverse sun damage in the outer skin-cell layer. Nonprescription vitamin C products are also helpful.

Another treatment consists of a peel that contains two topical solutions used together–the Jessner solution, an alpha hydroxy peeling solution, and Efudex, an anti–sun damage medicine. The peels are performed as a series of eight weekly treatments. First, the Jessner solution goes on, then the Efudex, which is left on the skin. The beauty of this treatment is that it results in little redness or peeling.

Collagen injections by a dermatologist or a plastic surgeon can help plump up sagging skin that has lost its support.

Q: How can I fight under-eye bags?

A: The skin under eyes and on lids can get puffy from a multitude of evils: alcohol, allergies, crying, and/or salt consumption. Prevent this by sleeping with your head propped up (fluid tends to pool under your eyes when your head is level with your body). When it comes to under-eye treatments, make sure they contain key antioxidants, such as vitamins A, C, and E.

Q: Can you shrink large pores?

A: No. Your pores don't change size. Once a pore is stretched, it can never fully close, but it can appear smaller by cleansing it of sebum and dirt. Moisturizers hydrate skin, making pores appear smaller against moisture-filled skin. Masks and astringents mildly irritate the face, causing skin to puff up around pores, making them look smaller. An astringent that contains ingredients like witch hazel, aluminum salts, lactic acid, and citric acid can help shrink pores temporarily. Also try pore-cleansing strips, which adhere to the skin and are then pulled away, at the same time pulling away pore-clogging oil and dirt. Pore treatments to try include Bioré Self-Heating Moisture Mask, Almay's StayClean Medicated Pore Strips, and Elizabeth Arden's Pore-Fix C.

Q: I have back acne. What can I do?

A: Wash your back daily with a gentle-bristled scrub brush. For blackheads and little red bumps, wash with a mild, salicyclic acid cleanser, such as SalAc Wash. Also dab on a 2.5 to 10 percent benzoyl peroxide treatment (if skin is oily and not irritated, you can go to 10 percent). But don't try scrubbing and applying benzoyl peroxide on serious acne—any large, red, or painful cysts need to be looked at by your dermatologist. Also, take care using benzoyl peroxide, because it can bleach clothing it comes into contact with.

Q: I've been breaking out on my décolletage. What should I do?

A: The skin on your upper chest, or décolletage, is very delicate, and that area contains fewer sebaceous glands than the face. Consequently, oil and sweat can build up, especially after workouts, resulting in chest pimples. If you get breakouts, wash with a mild, antibacterial soap. Then, treat pimples with an over-the-counter 2.5 percent (if skin is very oily, 10 percent) benzoyl peroxide product that's tinted to cover as it heals (try Neutrogena On-the-Spot Acne Treatment Cream). Follow with an oil-free facial moisturizer, or use an AHA cream to keep skin clean, clear, and protected (such as Purpose, Neutrogena, Eucerin, or L'Oréal Plenitude Excell-A3 Cream with SPF 8).

Q: How can I tame my rough elbows and knees?

A: Got rough spots there? You're not alone. The skin's top layer of dead cells (the stratum corneum) is thicker on knees and elbows, because these parts get bumped and chafed constantly. Apply a good moisturizer with urea, salicylic acid, or an alpha hydroxy acid. If skin becomes cracked and painful, get a super-sloughing, 12 percent AHA product (now available over-the-counter as Am-Lactin, or the prescription Lac-Hydrin). If that doesn't help, see your dermatologist.

Q: What can I do about pimples on my buttocks?

A: Little bumps popping out on your butt? This can result from tight-fitting clothes, which can slow the skin's natural exfoliating process and lead to bump buildup. Normally, bacteria sit on the skin, but tight-fitting clothing can rub the bacteria back down into the pores,

> ### *Quick Tip*
>
> Want to stop looking in the mirror and seeing puffy eyes come the A.M.? Sleep with your head elevated on two pillows. This prevents fluid from accumulating in your face as you sleep, by allowing it to drain away from your head through your bloodstream.

causing breakouts. Plus, your normal sweat provides a moist breeding ground on which bacteria can proliferate. To fix: wear looser-fitting clothing and wash with an antibacterial soap, such as Dial, Lever 2000, or Oilatum AD. Another remedy is to avoid using any fabric softeners in the dryer, because the fibers left on your underwear can further irritate your skin. Use an AHA lotion to speed exfoliation.

Q: What's the best way to prevent foot odor?

A: Sprinkle baking soda over clean feet to soak up perspiration and to control smell. You can also sprinkle it inside shoes. Also, opt for leather shoes over man-made fibers as well as cotton socks rather than acrylic, since leather shoes and cotton socks absorb perspiration and allow the feet to breathe. Try Zeasorb-AF powder, which is an over-the-counter drying and antifungal preparation.

Q: Should you trim your cuticles during each manicure?

A: Cutting cuticles leaves edges split and ragged, increasing the risk of bacterial and yeast infections. You can also damage the nail bed permanently. Many people do clip their cuticles, and most experience no problems. However, the ones who end up in my office are those that have contracted bacterial or yeast infections under and/or around the nails. The cuticle's sole purpose in life is to provide a barrier for that part of the finger from water and other bacteria. If you tend to get infections, nix the clippers and opt, instead, for using a cuticle softener or moisturizing cream before pushing back cuticles with either an orangewood stick or the edge of a towel wrapped around your finger. Another option: cuticle remover. But be careful: many cuticle removers contain sodium hydroxide, a caustic chemical that can destroy skin tissue and cause irritation if left on for too long.

Q: Is the best intensive conditioner for dry, damaged hair a hot oil treatment?

A: Used for centuries, hot oil treatments coat the hair shaft, making it lank. An effective conditioner should contain protein and moisture. Oil and water don't mix—and oil doesn't contain protein. Protein acts like plaster to fill in cracks and to smooth the hair shaft, making it stronger. Oil, on the other hand, has a molecular structure that is too large to penetrate into the hair. The result: oil sits on top of the hair, making it flat; conditioners that contain some oil work, because the small amount of oil they contain lubricates and smoothes the cuticle. For maximum benefit, apply conditioner, then cover hair with a warm towel (heat opens up the hair cuticle, allowing the conditioner to penetrate).

Q: Do the best exfoliators have tiny, dry particles in them?

A: Although they may feel like they're working, exfoliators of this type can actually scratch and abrade the skin. Avoid products containing sharp, hard particles, especially natural ingredients, such as ground walnut shells, apricot seeds, and oatmeal, because all can cause microscopic tears in the skin. Some companies are forsaking natural grains for smooth, synthetic spherical beads. For maximum benefit: gently massage scrub into wet skin for three minutes and rinse with tepid water.

Q: Which "miracle" creams, lotions, and cosmetics can permanently reduce the signs of aging?

A: Don't buy this bill of goods! The FDA is having a field day with companies that claim their products slow down or completely erase the effects of aging. According to a set of cosmetic guidelines established by Congress more than fifty years ago, any product that intends to alter the function or structure of skin is a drug and must undergo rigorous testing that can take up to 10 years.

Very often "miracle" treatments will contain the latest revolutionary ingredients: bee pollen, turtle oil, collagen, elastin, hormones, placenta–none of which have been proven to work permanently. So far, no one has found a way to reverse the signs of aging, by any means other than plastic surgery, collagen injections, vitamin A treatments, alpha hydroxy acids, chemical peels, cosmetic surgery, dermabrasion, or Botox.

Q: Should you apply alcohol to oily skin to reduce oil?

A: Never. Alcohol dehydrates skin's upper layers and alters its pH balance, leaving it susceptible to breakouts. In fact, it may cause glands to work harder to replace the lost oil.

Q: How can I take care of my lips, so they don't chap?

A: To soothe dry, possibly chapped lips, slick on a lip protector. Follow with just a dab of a lip-toned lipstick for the most natural look

---

Quick Tip

Lavender gets its name from *lavare*, the Latin word meaning "to bathe." Ancient Romans used the herb to scent their baths.

Did you know that...

In the Middle Ages, when smooth skin was seen as a sign of purity, women plucked their eyebrows and their hairlines to appear virtuous.

possible. Be careful about the lipstick you use. Matte lipsticks, which lack certain moisturizing ingredients, tend to leave lips parched–especially in cold weather. The same holds for lip balms that contain phenol, which also can be too drying. A better choice: lip gloss or a cream-based lipstick fortified with aloe, mineral oil, or vitamin E (try Cabot's). To keep lips smooth, always wear lip balm on its own or under your lipstick. Look for a balm loaded with emollients, such as petrolatum, lanolin, and cocoa butter. Balms work in two ways: they create a barrier against the harsh elements, and they seal in moisturizer.

Q: What are all these blotches and splotches on my face, and how can I get rid of them?

A: Brown spots and freckles are caused by the sun. Either you haven't always worn sunscreen, or your sun sensitivity is heightened due to an increase in estrogen from birth-control pills or pregnancy. Future spots are preventable with sunscreen, but to tackle the ones you've got, try incorporating into your routine AHAs or a cream from the vitamin A family. Hydroquinone is also an effective bleaching agent (found over-the-counter in Bioelements Pigment Discourager as well as in the by-prescription products Lustra AF, Eldoquin, and Melenex). A word of warning: in darker skins, hydroquinone may create the opposite effect of making skin even darker. New skin lighteners containing botanical extracts combined with vitamin C and AHAs eliminate that problem. Red areas are usually blood vessels showing through the skin, a form of rosacea. The causes are almost anything that makes skin flush: alcohol, spicy food, exercise, sun exposure. Over time, the vessels become permanently dilated. Trying to avoid some of these sources is one way to calm your color. A doctor can also prescribe topical or oral antibiotics that can diminish redness.

Q: What can I do for hair loss?

A: Stress is often a key cause of hair loss. Here's what happens: The blood vessels constrict, depriving the hair follicles of the oxygen, minerals, and vitamins they need for healthy hair growth. Vitamins are depleted when you are under stress, because the body burns more energy and directs nutrients and vitamins to those parts that need it for survival–like the heart, lungs, and brain. For that reason, and under those conditions, the scalp will not get the benefit of these essential nutrients. To solve the problem:

- Take 2.5 milligrams of biotin orally each day. (Biotin is a water-soluble vitamin–meaning, what you don't use, you excrete–that is essential for hair and nail growth.)
- Some women can experience hair loss because they are not getting enough protein in their diets. You should aim to eat protein like chicken, fish, lean meat, beans, nuts, and seeds, milk, yogurt, and cheese. It's also essential to take a good daily multi-vitamin and a B-complex vitamin.
- Use products containing B5 panthenol to strengthen the hair shaft and to plump up the hair by building up the cuticle from within.
- Wash with volumizing shampoos, which usually contain keratin or protein to build up the hair shaft.
- If any of the above solutions don't work, you may want to check with your doctor, since hair loss can be a symptom of a medical condition.

Q: I'm only 23, so why is my hair so gray?

A: Occasionally, premature gray hair signals a thyroid problem. It's easy to find out by asking your doctor for a blood test to check it out. If the results indicate you have an underactive thyroid–meaning the gland doesn't produce enough of the hormone thyroxine–the problem can be corrected with a prescription for thyroid hormone replacement. Otherwise, there's not much you can do about early graying, since it's probably an inherited condition. Gray hair occurs when cells at the base of your hair follicles stop producing a pigment called melanin. The good news: earlier scares about hair dye being a possible cause of cancer have not been proved, so it's safe to cover the gray. And perhaps soon there will be a medical way to permanently reverse the gray. Scientists reportedly have found a way to deliver melanin to hair follicles in tests, turning white-haired mice black.

Q: What is atopic dermatitis? Is it the same as eczema?

A: The word eczema is used to describe all kinds of red, blistering, oozing, scaly, brownish, thickened, and itching skin conditions. Atopic dermatitis is one kind of common eczema, which can run in families, often occurring in infants and young children. It's an itchy rash of inflamed skin. Although atopic dermatitis is associated with allergies, it's usually not triggered by any foods. It can be treated externally with medicated creams or ointments and can be prevented somewhat by keeping the skin well hydrated and moisturized.

Myth:

If you pluck out a gray hair, 10 more will grow in its place.

FACT:

Plucking out a gray hair will not make 10 more grow back. Instead, just one hair will grow back, which also will most likely be gray. The reason is, the pigment-producing cells at the hair follicle are probably worn out. It doesn't matter whether you shave, pluck, or wax the hair; none of these methods has any effect on how the hair will grow back. And, by the way, the hair will not grow back darker or coarser (another myth). That's because the different kinds of hair that grow on your body (eyebrows versus hair on your head versus pubic hair) are genetically programmed to grow a certain color at a certain rate at a certain texture. As anyone who has ever struggled with trying to permanently remove unwanted hair knows, trying to change nature's course is not easy.

Q: I have a tiny little growth on the side of my neck. It doesn't hurt but it annoys me. What could this be?

A: It sounds like a skin tag, a small overgrowth of normal skin that protrudes from the skin. They usually occur in areas of friction like underarms, groin, and under breasts, and appear as we age, as a normal part of the aging process. They also tend to appear during pregnancy and after weight gain. They run in the family, are 100 percent harmless, and can be removed by having them either surgically snipped off or cauterized. Of course, like other spots on the body, if they change color or begin to bleed, have your dermatologist check them out.

Q: I've noticed little red dots sprinkled on my body, arms, and legs. What are they?

A: They are called cherry angiomas and are dilated "broken" blood vessels that are slightly raised and red. They are completely harmless, and most Caucasians get them as a part of getting older. Like skin tags, cherry angiomas tend to run in families. They can be removed by surgical snipping, cauterizing, or laser.

Q: What can I do to help alleviate the itching from my poison ivy rash without a prescription?

A: Dip a washcloth in cool milk and place it over the rash to soothe the itch and inflammation of poison ivy. You can also get an over-the-counter 1 percent cortisone cream.

Q: I have an itchy rash under my arms. What can I do about it?

A: Stop using deodorant, and wash the area with fragrance-free Dove. Then apply good old-fashioned Arm & Hammer baking soda under your arms after showering for the next one to two weeks.

Q: I had a wart treated by my doctor, but it came back. What do I do now?

A: Warts are a non-cancerous skin growth caused by a viral infection in the top layer of the skin. They can be stubborn and may need several treatments before they disappear, sometimes only to reappear somewhere else. Warts should be treated as they appear to help prevent them from spreading. They are not usually dangerous (except in the case of genital warts in women, which can lead to cervical cancer), but they can be painful, especially if they are on the soles of the feet (plantar warts). Keep your follow-up appointments with your doctor and use any at-home medications regularly until your doctor says treatment is no longer necessary.

Q: After I used my new tangerine shower gel, I got a rash. Am I allergic?

A: Not necessarily. It may just be an irritation, the common response to super scented products (especially during cold-weather months, when skin is drier and therefore more sensitive). Unless you've got red bumps or hives (red, itchy patches), assume your skin is just irritated. Stop using the product immediately and apply an over-the-counter 1 percent cortisone ointment (like Hytone) to the area.

If redness and itching don't disappear within a week, contact a dermatologist, who can determine whether you've got an allergy by examining the rash and discussing the products you use. (You can develop an allergy to products you've been using for a while.) Your doctor may need to do a patch test to evaluate your skin's reaction to test strips of common chemical and fragrance allergens. Either way, it's best to give your skin a break and stick to a fragrance-free product (like Cetaphil Liquid cleanser). But beware: all unscented products aren't necessarily fragrance-free; in fact, they can contain a masking scent that covers up the smell of the ingredients and can still damage sensitive skin.

Q: I have these awful-looking, thick, dry patches on my elbows, and no amount of moisturizer seems to improve them. Could it be something "medical"?

A: You may have psoriasis, a persistent skin disease in which the skin is inflamed with dry, silver-colored scales. The cause is unknown, but psoriasis can run in families and can be activated by infections such as strep throat. It appears most commonly on the elbows, knees, arms, legs, scalp, and nails. It can be treated with prescription medications to loosen the scales and stop itching. Controlled exposure to sunlight or medically supervised ultraviolet light therapy is also used.

Did you know that...

To achieve the pale complexion popular in eighteenth-century Europe, women ate wafers that contained the poison arsenic.

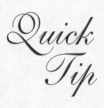

To conceal a cold sore:

- Using a damp cosmetic sponge, apply regular foundation mixed with a few drops of moisturizer directly onto the cold sore.
- Blend well.
- Throw out the sponge.
- Apply lip balm to lips.
- Apply lipstick with a cotton tip (to avoid reinfecting yourself).

Q: My face lately seems to be always red and breaking out, especially on my cheeks and chin. Should I be using Retin-A?

A: It sounds like you may have rosacea, a condition affecting the skin of the face. Rosacea usually starts with redness on the cheeks and can slowly worsen to include one or more additional symptoms, including acne, on other parts of the face. The redness usually looks like blushing or a sunburn, often combined with small, red pimples (papules). Small blood vessels in the face may become pronounced, and if the condition goes untreated, knobby bumps may appear on the nose. Although rosacea cannot be cured, it can be controlled by topical and oral medications as well as by minimizing the causes of flushing and blushing, which can lead to rosacea flares. Avoiding rosacea "triggers," such as hot and spicy foods, alcohol, extreme heat or cold, and stress, can help reduce rosacea exacerbations. Use gentle cleansers, along with a daily sunscreen of at least SPF 15 as well as continued treatment with prescribed medications.

Q: My eyebrows are dry and flaky, almost like dandruff. Is this just dry skin?

A: It could be seborrheic dermatitis, an inflammation in areas having the greatest number of sebaceous oil glands of the skin (like the scalp, sides of the nose, and behind the ears). The area may appear red and crusty or flaky. Seborrheic dermatitis is not uncommon, especially in people with lighter skin, nor is it harmful. In infants, it is called "cradle cap." It cannot be prevented, but it can be treated successfully with medicated shampoos and topical prescription medications.

Q: I have a rash. How can I tell what it's from?

A: Many rashes are a contact dermatitis, meaning that the rash is caused by a reaction to something the skin has come into contact with. The substance can be either an irritant or an allergen.

An irritant is something that almost anyone would get a reaction to, such as a very harsh chemical, whereas an allergen will cause a reaction only in susceptible individuals (for example, if you get a reaction to poison ivy).

Common allergens include nickel (found in jewelry and metal objects), rubber, dyes, preservatives, fragrances, and poison ivy and related plants.

Your dermatologist can perform a patch test, which involves taping a panel infused with common allergens onto your skin and seeing if any particular substance causes a reaction.

Q: I told my father not to kiss the grandchildren while he has a cold sore on his lip, but he doesn't believe me that they are contagious. Are they?

A: You're right: Cold sores, or herpes simplex virus type 1, are contagious by kissing or by using the same eating utensils or towels. The sores, which occur shortly after exposure, most commonly affect the lips, mouth, nose, chin, or cheeks. A primary infection lasts from seven to 10 days, with the sores appearing as tiny, clear, fluid-filled blisters that eventually break, crust, and then heal. The virus, however, remains in the body in a dormant phase, living in the nerves. Illness, sun exposure, or stress can trigger recurrent outbreaks—or, the sores may never recur at all. There is no vaccine to prevent or cure this disease, but recurrent outbreaks can be controlled by taking oral medication when the patient feels an outbreak coming on (this is indicated by tingling, burning, itching, or tenderness in the area where the outbreak usually occurs). Because ultraviolet light damages fibers in the immune system, it's a good idea, if you suffer from cold sores, to protect your lips with an ultraviolet-protective lip balm when you are in the sun.

Myth:

You have to kiss someone on the lips to get their cold sore or fever blister.

FACT:

Yes and no. You must come into direct contact with the virus causing the cold sores or fever blisters—which certainly can happen from kissing the affected person, but also from many other points of contact. You can also get it by using the same eating utensils, towels, or lip balm. Cold sores and fever blisters are not caused by a cold or fever; they are common names for herpes simplex virus type 1. The type 2 herpes virus causes genital sores, and is most often transmitted through sexual contact with an infected person.

chapter six

Problem Solved

*You can complain because roses have thorns, or you
can rejoice because thorns have roses.*
—ZIGGY

IN CENTURIES AND EVEN DECADES PAST, MANY WOMEN WOULD NEVER HAVE DREAMED of discussing their "real women" problem areas with each other, much less with a doctor. Instead, they relied on old wives' potions and lotions, and often they were lucky to escape with their lives, let alone get rid of their skin/body problems. Thankfully, times have changed. Today women speak to each other and to their doctors about topics such as dark areas of pigmentation, circles under the eyes, moles, excess hair, mustaches, spider veins, and stretch marks. This chapter explores the most common complaints I hear from my patients and the beauty editors of the magazines that call me for guidance, plus the easiest, most cost-effective (and longest-lasting) solutions. If something bothers you about your body, now you can take steps to change it based on solid, medically sound information without grasping in the dark for just any old solution.

What Do I Do About Dark Spots on My Face?

I find that women complain about two main types of darkened, or pigmented, areas on their skin. The first, freckles (or lentigines), are fairly well-defined, easy-to-recognize, circular areas of increased pigmentation. Many women (and men) don't mind freckles and often find that other people think they are quite attractive, especially when sprinkled across the bridge of the nose and across the cheeks.

The other type of pigmentation—large patches of increased color called melasma— is another story. Melasma areas differ from freckles in that they are much less clearly defined and are often quite larger than freckles. Also, unlike freckles, melasma is due to hormonal fluctuations, which is why it often occurs during pregnancy and when a woman is on the birth control pill or hormone replacement therapy. It results when estrogen hormones stimulate the production of melanin (pigment), resulting in splotchy patches of increased pigmentation. Essentially, the hormone-sensitized cells are tanning, but at a faster rate than the surrounding skin. Most women hate it when these dark patches appear on the face, usually above the lip, on the forehead, and along the temples.

Removing Dark Spots and Splotches

Both freckles and melasma are due in part to ultraviolet exposure. So, to avoid both kinds of excess pigmentation, you must ensure that you adequately protect yourself from sun exposure. The sun hits us with two main wavelengths of ultraviolet light: ultraviolet A (UVA) and ultraviolet B (UVB). Most sunscreens have an SPF rating that protects primarily against UVB rays; fewer sunscreens protect against UVA. Although UVA is considered a weaker ultraviolet radiation, it, too, can cause increased color pigmentation. That's why it's essential for you to choose a sunscreen or blocking agent that protects against both UVB and UVA light (such as Parsol 1789, zinc oxide, or titanium dioxide).

Besides preventative measures, you can use a lightening agent, such as hydroquinone, in a 4 percent solution to help reduce the pigmentation. Hydroquinone comes in several different formulations. The one I recommend most often is Lustra AF, which combines the 4 percent hydroquinone with Parsol 1789, as well as with glycolic acid and topical vitamin C. Another effective method for fading both freckles and melasma is vitamin A–based topicals, such as one of my personal favorites, Avita cream. This cream contains tretinoin, the same active ingredient as in Retin-A, but in a far milder formulation, or base, that doesn't irritate your skin as traditional Retin-A therapy does.

I recommend you avoid using natural remedies, like lemon or lime juice, on your freckles to fade them. These juices contain natural photosensitizers and may only make skin more prone to darkening.

Freckles can also be treated with cryosurgery, a process by which a dermatologist applies liquid nitrogen to the skin. The treated skin forms a scab and falls off. Another method of removing freckles is called electrodesiccation. In this procedure, a clinician touches the freckle with a needle that emits an electric spark, destroying the cell's pigment, which causes the freckle to fade away.

With melasma, estrogen stimulates the pigment-producing sites, making these areas especially sensitive to ultraviolet light. Consequently, the cells respond quickly to any sun exposure and darken faster than the surrounding skin cells. No one knows exactly why this occurs, but if you have this problem, you might want to discontinue taking birth-control pills, because of the added estrogen in the pills.

If the lightening agents don't work, then you may want to try a series of glycolic facial treatments (10 to 70 percent solutions), amino fruit acid treatments, or microdermabrasion treatments. Any of these procedures will help to remove increased pigmentation from the skin. In extreme cases of freckling, laser resurfacing with the erbium or, possibly, the carbon dioxide lasers may also work well (see Chapter 14). Carbon dioxide is riskier for darker skin types because it can affect color more than the other modalities.

You can also end up with darker areas on your skin when acne, a cut, or a rash heals. This is called postinflammatory hyperpigmentation; these dark spots take about six months to fade away naturally.

Mole Alert: Which Ones Need to Be Removed?

People occasionally worry unnecessarily about moles. For example, it's a fact that most people will produce new moles up to the age of 40 or 45. Based on that, if you are under the age of, say, 50 and develop a new mole, it is not necessarily suspicious. Now, if you are 70 and discover a new mole, that should definitely be grounds for suspicion.

Get-Rid-of-It Guidelines

If you are looking for guidelines, The American Academy of Dermatology (www.aad.org) publishes what are known as the A, B, C, D, E criteria for the evaluation of moles:

A = Asymmetry. Is the mole symmetrical, meaning of equal proportion in size and shape (normal), or asymmetrical, of unequal proportions (suspicious)?

B = Border. Does the mole have an even, well-defined border (normal) or an irregular border (suspicious)?

C = Color. Is the mole one homogeneous color (normal unless dark brown or black) or multiple colors (suspicious)?

D = Diameter. Does the mole measure less than (normal) or more than (suspicious) 6 millimeters (.6 centimeters), about one-third of an inch, in diameter?

E = Elevated. Is the surface of the mole flat (normal) or elevated (suspicious)?

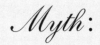

Myth:

You can get a healthy tan.

FACT:

If you're getting a tan, you are doing damage. Tanning is the body's response to injury by the sun's ultraviolet radiation. What's worse than sun exposure? Exposure to the UVA rays in tanning booths. UVA rays penetrate even deeper into the skin than UVB rays. The result: although damage isn't visible to the naked eye (as with sunburn caused by UVB rays), UVA rays cause greater damage to collagen. You can also develop skin and eye irritations, allergic reactions, and premature aging.

Types of Moles

Once a month give yourself a complete skin check after you've taken a shower. If you see a mole you haven't noticed before, ask yourself whether the mole in question looks like anything else on your body. If it does, it is probably not a skin cancer, or melanoma. It is extremely rare for a person to have multiple skin malignancies; therefore if you can find a mole or, even better, a few moles that look similar in appearance to the new mole, you can be more certain the mole is not cancerous. If the mole does not appear to match any other mole on your body, that doesn't necessarily mean it's malignant, but it does mean you need your dermatologist to check it out. The other thing to watch out for is a mole that has changed in one or more of the following ways: raised; grown in size; changed color; developed irregularities in the border; become itchy, irritated, and/or bleeding. Again, the emergence of these characteristics doesn't necessarily mean you have cancer, but you do need a dermatologist to check out any moles that have recently changed, just to make sure. If you follow these simple rules, I believe you'll stay out of trouble 99 percent of the time. And if you discover a mole that fits any of the above criteria, you're better off having it removed and tested, so you can find out what's wrong in time to do something about it.

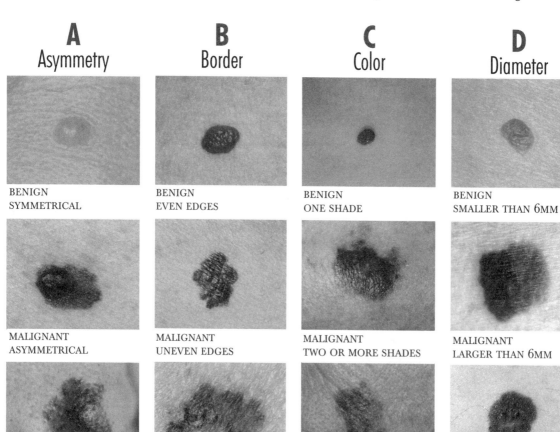

A Asymmetry	**B** Border	**C** Color	**D** Diameter
BENIGN SYMMETRICAL	BENIGN EVEN EDGES	BENIGN ONE SHADE	BENIGN SMALLER THAN 6MM
MALIGNANT ASYMMETRICAL	MALIGNANT UNEVEN EDGES	MALIGNANT TWO OR MORE SHADES	MALIGNANT LARGER THAN 6MM
MALIGNANT ASYMMETRICAL	MALIGNANT UNEVEN EDGES	MALIGNANT TWO OR MORE SHADES	MALIGNANT LARGER THAN 6MM

What Can I Do for Dark Circles under My Eyes?

At their worst, these dark, hollowed-out-looking circles can make you look like a cross between a raccoon and a femme fatale suffering from consumption. At best, they make you look really tired. Dark circles under the eyes are really a combination of sun damage and blood flow from the capillaries in this area. It's also genetic (if your mother or father had them, you're likely to have them too). Because your eyelid skin is the thinnest skin in the body, sun damage shows up quickly here in the form of dilating and increased blood flow to the area. As a result, you can see a dark glow or color through the transparency of the skin.

Several treatments work to lessen under-eye circles by lightening the pigmentation that has accumulated from sun damage. For starters, you may want to use a lightening agent, such as hydroquinone, in conjunction with an alpha hydroxy agent, something from the vitamin A family, and a sunscreen. You'll need to be patient, because, depending on the severity of the pigmentation or circles, it can easily take up to six months to see any kind of improvement.

If your dark circles are very severe, I recommend in-office treatments with either glycolic acid, amino fruit acid, or microdermabrasion (see Chapter 11). For the most extreme cases, I recommend laser therapy; if it involves a vascular component (broken blood vessels), I suggest a pulsed dye laser. If it involves sun pigmentation, I suggest a resurfacing laser such as erbium or carbon dioxide.

Test to Determine a Vascular Problem

Look in the mirror and push down on the area with your finger and gently move it across the skin. If you see that the area is lighter and clearer while you are pressing on it, then you have a broken blood vessel, indicating a vascular component, which requires a pulsed dye laser. What happens is, when you press on the skin, you squeeze the blood out and down, which makes the whole area appear lighter. If you see no change in coloration when you push down on the area, then the dark circles don't include a blood component, and a resurfacing laser is needed.

What Can I Do for Broken Blood Vessels?

Broken blood vessels can appear anywhere on the body, but are most commonly found on the face, neck, and legs. They are simply dilated skin blood vessels. Once they are visible through the skin, the only way to get rid of them is to obliterate them—by laser, if they're on the face, or by injection or laser, if they show up on the body. Once zapped, they are reabsorbed by the body.

You're most likely to find broken blood vessels on the head and neck, and on the legs, where they show up in the form of tiny spider veins. When you discover these little broken blood vessels, stop yourself from rushing off to buy a cream that is touted as being able to reduce or eliminate broken blood vessels; all it will reduce is your bank account. As of today, no cream can impact these capillaries.

Zapping Broken Facial Capillaries

Most physicians recommend using lasers to zap broken blood vessels on the face. I normally recommend the pulsed dye laser, because I believe it's the most effective at clearing broken capillaries. Here's how it works: the wavelength of light is absorbed by the red blood cells inside the selected vessels, heating up the cells, which then disintegrate the surrounding blood vessels. The only downside of this laser is that it leaves you with some purple bruising at the site of the treatment area, which lasts a few days to a week and can be difficult to camouflage with makeup. I recommend you consult with your doctor to determine which laser best suits your needs, taking into consideration the effectiveness of the laser for your problem as well as your individual recovery needs and the recovery period for the laser treatment.

The Line on Leggy Spider Veins

Many women have told me of the misery of discovering unattractive blue and red spider veins on their legs, just as they were heading out to the beach sporting a sexy, new bathing suit. What causes those mottled little lines on your legs? They occur for a number of reasons. They are hereditary; if your mother has spider veins, you are likely to eventually get them too. Women who spend lots of time on their feet are likely to develop spider veins, because the pressure on the area forces the veins to fill up with blood and protrude. If you are overweight, bingo—another cause of spider veins. Another reason spider veins can develop is due to increased levels of estrogen. That's why pregnancy, taking birth control pills, and hormone replacement therapy can result in an increase in spider veins.

If you are one of the millions of women who have spider veins, the best way to get rid of them is to have sclerotherapy injections combined with compression. Although this can take many forms, in my practice I usually have patients wear compression-grade stockings 24 hours a day for three days immediately following the injections and then just during the day for another several days to a week following injections.

A sclerotherapy treatment consists of injecting a solution into the veins, which immediately dissolves them without injuring the surrounding area. Most patients require two to four treatments at approximately four-week intervals between treatments.

Laser therapy is another popular method used to erase unsightly spider veins. However, I usually recommend sclerotherapy as my first-choice treatment, because the laser procedure produces several negative effects, including bruising and changes in pigmentation that can linger for months. The only time I do recommend using lasers for treating spider veins is when the spider veins are very, very tiny—too small to inject with the sclerotherapy solution.

Removing Varicose Veins

Varicose veins are abnormally swollen or enlarged blood vessels that occur when the wall of the vein weakens. When this happens, the swollen vessels can cause leg pain. In the past, the only way to get rid of these defective, varicose, veins was by surgically stripping them away. But in March 1999, the Food and Drug Administration approved a new, minimally invasive procedure for treating varicose veins, called the closure technique, that can be performed in a doctor's office. The technique, which is not yet widely available in the U.S., involves inserting a small tube, called a catheter, into the defective vein through a small puncture. The catheter delivers radio frequency energy to the vein wall, causing the vein to shrink and seal shut. Once the diseased vein is closed, neighboring healthy veins take over to restore normal outflow of blood from the legs. Patients experience minimal bruising and recover quickly.

Ambulatory phlebectomy is another new technique for removing larger varicose veins; it, too, causes minimal bruising and can usually be done in one treatment. First, large varicose veins near the surface of the skin are marked with a special light source, making the vein dark against a light background, so it's easier to see. Then, a local anesthetic is injected alongside and under the vein being removed. Next, a series of small needle punctures is made, through which portions of the varicose vein are then gently pulled using a special instrument.

Can Anything Remove Stretch Marks?

Often, the first time you notice stretch marks on your body is when you're pregnant or after you've just lost or gained considerable weight.

Basically, stretch marks appear when the skin is stretched or distended, such as during growth spurts, workouts, and, of course, pregnancy. Rapid and extensive stretching or distending of the skin breaks down the skin's collagen and elastin fibers faster than they can reproduce or elongate. Like little springs, these fibers expand to the point of no return, then they snap. Stretch marks typically look like uneven layers of pigmentation in the skin, because with stretch marks, the normal thin top layer of skin sits on top of an uneven and fragmented support structure (the dermis), where the collagen and elastin proteins are located.

First, the good news: stretch marks are not harmful to your skin's health. Now, the bad news: no perfect treatment exists for stretch marks, and nobody knows why some women get them and others don't. Although no currently available treatment can completely remove stretch marks, several treatments are available to help improve the appearance of stretch marks.

A Torrent of Stretch Mark Treatments

Several fairly effective methods are used to treat stretch marks, although none of them are perfect. All treatment methods work better on relatively new stretch marks with a pinkish tint than on older marks that have turned white.

Treatments for stretch marks include applying topical products, such as alpha hydroxy acids and derivatives of vitamin A (Retin-A, Renova, Avita, Differin, Tazorac) as well as a number of more sophisticated in-office procedures. The current gold standard in-office treatment for stretch marks is treating them with the pulsed dye laser, the same procedure used to treat broken blood vessels and certain types of scars (see Chapter 14). This laser zaps stretch marks when the beam of light activates cells, called fibroblasts, into producing collagen and elastin, which replace the damaged collagen and elastin. The only side effect is a slightly bruised appearance to the stretch marks, which fades within a few days to a couple of weeks. You'll need one to three rounds of pulsed dye laser treatments to see improvement, and you should schedule the treatments six to 12 weeks apart to allow the skin time to heal.

In-office glycolic acid or microdermabrasion treatments can help with a 6- to 12- session course, but they aren't as effective as the pulsed dye laser treatment, which is, as I said, the gold standard.

What doesn't work as well? Over-the-counter preparations, such as cocoa butter.

How Can I Get Rid of Excess Hair?

A lot of treatments are available for removing excess hair, including mustaches and other facial hair as well as hair on the arms, breasts, stomach, thighs, calves, bikini area, and, especially for men, hair on the back and the back of the neck. If you have any of these problems, you must first figure out whether you are dealing with a hormonal problem, in which case, you'd need to see an endocrinologist.

It's fairly easy to tell if your problem is hormonal. Women with hormonal abnormalities often have an irregular menstrual cycle, or a very heavy flow, as well as severe cystic acne.

The more common cause of excess body and facial hair is genetics. Check out the hairiness of your relatives; if they sprout lots of hair in similar places, you probably inherited that propensity as well. One sign that your condition is genetic and not hormonal: the hair looks like your other hair and is distributed evenly all over the body. If you have any doubts as to which category you fit into, you should see your doctor before starting any method of treatment.

The ways to treat excess growth include shaving, waxing, tweezing, electrolysis (see Chapter 13), and using lasers and other light sources (see Chapter 14).

Radiant Treatment

Currently, several lasers have proven to be highly effective at reducing hair growth. These include the diode laser, the ruby laser, the alexandrite laser, and the broad spectrum light source, which is not technically a laser. These systems all work by targeting the melanin pigment in the hair and hair follicles. Unfortunately, none of these treatments take out all of the hair follicles in one shot; you'll need several treatments to achieve an 80 to 90 percent reduction.

Hair's Growing Pains

All hair follicles undergo a growth cycle. During the active growing stage (anagen), the hair is large and heavily pigmented, creating a ready-made, highly visible target for any of the lasers or light sources. During the resting stage (telogen), the hair looks thin and colorless, making it virtually invisible to the laser or light source used to treat it. That's why getting rid of excess hair usually requires several treatments, allowing for four- to eight-week intervals between each treatment, so you can catch the follicles during the (anagen) growing stage.

For the lasers to do their job properly, at the time of treatment the hair needs to be close to the skin's surface, not sticking out. Otherwise, the laser targets the hair, sitting on top of the skin, rather than the hair follicle.

You also should avoid waxing, tweezing, and plucking stray hairs before laser or light treatment, because you'll take out the hair root from the hair follicle, leaving no target for the laser or light source.

The Hairy No Tanning Rule

When lasering off hair, it's very important that you keep your skin as pale as possible (this means no tanning)! The reason you need to stay fair is that these systems not only target hair follicles, they also target melanin, or pigment. The last thing you want is to get rid of your excess hair only to be left with unsightly, uneven patches of discoloration on your skin.

The current laser and light therapies are wonderful, because they can treat most skin types and hair colors. The only exception to the rule is hair that is very, very gray-white or ultra blond, because those hair types contain virtually no melanin or pigment at all and therefore are harder to treat.

chapter seven

Hormones and the Life of Your Skin

If you can't change your fate, change your attitude.
—AMY TAN

HORMONES CAN BE TOUGH ON YOU. THEY WORK NIGHT AND DAY TO CONTROL physical and sexual activity; these chemical messengers also shake up your bodies from puberty, through menopause, and beyond. Although we have them to thank for making men men and women women, we also recognize that they can swing our moods, give us pimples, and make our hair go haywire. And that's only the beginning.

In this chapter, I'll cover some of your most common questions about how to deal with what your hormones do to your skin. It gives you a hormonal roadmap of your beauty needs (from menstruation to pregnancy and menopause) plus a skin shape-up program to chart your lifelong body and beauty changes from your twenties and beyond.

Q: How do hormones affect my acne?

A: Your hormones play a big factor in whether you develop acne. As a general rule, the hormone estrogen diminishes acne, while progesterone stimulates acne. That explains why women with "hormonal acne" tend to get flare-ups the week right before their menstrual cycle, following a spike in their progesterone levels. Taking birth control pills can help your acne, because the pills suppress and replace your own hormones with synthetic hormones, which are far less stimulating to the oil glands that cause acne flare-up. However, that is also why certain birth control pills may actually make acne worse—because the synthetic progesterone in the pill stimulates the oil glands as much as your own progesterone does.

75

Q: How does pregnancy affect my skin?

A: When it comes to your skin, the effects of pregnancy are often a throw of the dice. The skin of some women who had acne prior to getting pregnant clears completely and looks wonderful all the way through their pregnancies and postpartum periods. Other women who've never had a breakout before becoming pregnant may suddenly break out all over because of the tremendous hormonal changes that occur during pregnancy and immediately afterward. If that happens to you, first check with your doctor and then apply one of the following treatments, which are allowed by most OB/GYNs during pregnancy: topical benzoyl peroxides (as long as you're not allergic to them), in-office glycolic acid facials, and antibiotics (such as erythromycin) given topically or orally.

Program for Pregnant Women

- Wash with a mild cleanser (such as Dove or Cetaphil) twice daily.
- To open up blocked pores, exfoliate with an over-the-counter lotion containing glycolic or salicylic acid.
- Zap pimples with benzoyl peroxide. Try a 10 percent formula to dry up pimples and inhibit the growth of bacteria that cause new blemishes to form.
- Use oral antibiotics such as erythromycin, if first approved by your OB/GYN.

Q: How does hormone replacement therapy affect my skin?

A: When you use hormone replacement therapy (HRT), you basically add estrogen to the skin in the form of a patch or a cream. Estrogen leads to water retention, which is actually great for the skin, making it softer, more supple, and less dry and flaky. (The other side effect is that you get bloated more often, but consider it a tradeoff.) Scientists are at work trying to derive the same benefit in topical products for women who don't want to take hormone replacement therapy.

Q: Is sex good for my skin?

A: Sex is wonderful for the skin, just as it is wonderful for the rest of the body. And that's not just talk. In its most basic sense, sex releases feel-good endorphins, which make it a stress-reducing activity, a good cardiovascular workout, and ideally, a terrific emotional boost. This cocktail of positive influences is reflected in the skin's appearance—increasing blood flow throughout the body, causing you to have that rosy glow.

One caution to remember when cuddling: beard burn can cause trauma to the skin, resulting in breakouts. If you end up getting beard burn—red, irritated skin covered with little bumps—do the following: wash with an antiseptic soap (Oilatum AD, Lever 2000) and follow with a gentle moisturizer; if it's severe, use an over-the-counter 1 percent hydrocortisone cream. You might also be allergic to his aftershave or cologne, so watch out for that too.

Q: How does stress affect my skin?

A: We can't escape totally from stress. Whether we want to face it or not, stress is a part of our daily lives. Most of it comes from tiny moments that occur throughout the day: We get stuck in a traffic jam on the way to an important meeting; our sandwich is delivered without the right condiments; we spill coffee on our clothes just as we're walking out the door to a cocktail party. We may not even notice stress on a conscious level, but eventually we can't help but see its effects in the condition of our hair, skin, and nails. Stress does a huge number on our bodies, discharging stress hormones that increase blood pressure, raise pulse rates, and constrict blood vessels—effectively shunting blood away from the skin toward other organs. The sad result: muscles tense, and skin loses its rosy glow and begins to look wan and tired. If you don't have another reason to stop the chronic stress in your life, here's another wakeup call: as muscles tense under stress, you can begin to form fine lines and wrinkles. So, next time you get caught in a traffic jam, relax; you'll be doing your future face a favor.

Charting Your Hormones from Age 18 to 80

Your hormones follow a life cycle in your body. Let's explore how to deal with hormones as they change throughout your life from puberty, to PMS, through pregnancy, and menopause.

Don't Obsess Over PMS

About two weeks before menstruation begins, a woman's body steps up hormone production of estrogen and progesterone to prepare the uterus for possible pregnancy. At the same time, production of prostaglandins (hormone-like substances produced by the uterine lining that cause the uterus to relax and contract) increases. Skin problems can result when these hormones

Myth:

If I take Accutane (an acne drug), I may have problems bearing children.

FACT:

Taking Accutane does not compromise the future fertility or pregnancies of women of child-bearing years. However, if a female taking Accutane becomes pregnant, the fetus will almost certainly have birth defects. Taken as prescribed, with monthly visits to the dermatologist and careful blood monitoring, Accutane is a very safe and extremely effective drug for treating chronic, cystic acne. Some potential minor side effects are dryness of the skin, lips, and eyes, and muscle soreness.

rise, stimulating oil glands, clogging pores, and causing breakouts or acne. Stress further activates these glands. To prevent and combat blemishes:

* Wash daily with a gentle cleanser (such as Neutrogena), or use a mild soap for acne.
* Switch to a water-based foundation, which is less likely than oil-based makeup to clog pores.
* Use a clay-based mask to absorb excess oil from skin or try a gel mask containing benzoyl peroxide.
* Avoid getting a facial before or during your period. Most facials include massaging the skin, which makes acne worse by rupturing whiteheads under the skin.
* Your skin may feel extra-sensitive to pain just before your period. If so, hold off on tweezing and waxing during this time.

Will the Pill Make You Ill?

Several studies show that taking birth control pills can help reduce the bloating, depression, and irritability of PMS. Also, many doctors agree that the hormones in the pill protect women against ovarian cancer. Another plus: lower doses of hormones in the newer birth-control pills seem to reduce the risks of heart attacks, strokes, and blood clots associated with the older, higher-dosed pills. That's the good news. The bad news: taking the pill can open up a whole other can of worms. Here are some pill-related problems to watch out for and ways to deal with them:

Don't Sunbathe: Estrogen in the pill ups melanin production, but sometimes only in certain spots. So, when the sun hits the skin, those patches can get even darker.

Pimples? It could be the pill: If you're on the pill and struggle with acne, your choice of pill may be to blame. The hormone combinations in certain birth control pills (Ortho Tri-Cyclen, Ortho-Cyclen, Desogen, Demulen) may help acne; others may worsen it.

Scary Side Effects: More serious effects of birth control pills—such as depression or reduced sex drive—may require a change in the type of progesterone in the pill.

Hair Loss: Birth control pills are sometimes a factor in hair loss.

The Strain of Spider Veins: Estrogen causes blood vessels to dilate, causing little broken capillaries on the face as well as spider veins and varicose veins on the legs.

Pregnancy Problems

One of the most significant changes during pregnancy is the steep rise in estrogen levels, which typically kicks in about the sixth to tenth week and steadily rises throughout the pregnancy. Estrogen is responsible for that "glow," because it increases blood flow near the skin's surface. The hormone also reduces the production of sebum, which often makes it a boon to acne-ridden skin. However, it can also worsen acne, especially if you are undergoing more stress than normal.

Acne: You must exercise caution when treating acne during pregnancy and while nursing. Oral tetracycline, the antibiotic usually prescribed for cystic acne, can stain a developing baby's teeth. Also, Accutane, the vitamin A derivative often prescribed for acne, can cause birth defects, so you must not take it while pregnant or nursing. Your best bet is a topical antibiotic gel, cream, or liquid, an over-the-counter acne medication, or a series of glycolic acid facials. Many doctors advise pregnant women to stop using Retin-A or other topical vitamin A products until after they deliver. The reason is, they are made from vitamin A, which is toxic in large amounts.

Blotches and Growths: Because extra estrogen also affects the skin's pigmentation, you may get melasma, dark splotches on your upper cheeks, forehead, or upper lip (actually, an estimated 50 to 75 percent of pregnant women get melasma, which is often called "the mask of pregnancy"). Melasma is more common in darker-complexioned women, and it's also made worse by exposure to the sun's UV rays. Because the skin's pigmentation darkens with pregnancy, in addition to melasma, you may also develop darker nipples, and your birthmarks may deepen in color. Sometimes, skin tags–flesh-colored, benign growths–may appear on your body, and a dark vertical line may appear on your stomach. Good news: most of these all go away after you deliver the baby. Otherwise, a dermatologist can remove the growths. If the dark blotches don't leave, a dermatologist can use a hydroquinone solution of 4 percent to bleach them away.

Moles: Any existing moles on the body may grow slightly and get somewhat darker during pregnancy, which should cause no alarm. If a mole starts looking unusual in some other way (irregular borders, mottled coloring), see your doctor.

Stretch Marks: These are predetermined genetically (if your mother had stretch marks while pregnant, you are likely to get them too). The red lines are caused by the skin's stretching during the weight gain of pregnancy as well as by any rapid weight gain (including yo-yo dieting). Applying creams, cocoa butter, or vitamin E to the affected skin won't make stretch marks go away, unfortunately, but they can help alleviate the discomfort of itching and keep the skin smooth. Usually these marks lighten and fade with time. After you deliver, you can try some creams with vitamin A to slough off dead skin cells, which might help a little. Ultimately, however, the best way to attack stretch marks is with the pulsed dye laser, which stimulates collagen and elastin production without affecting the skin's surface, eliminating the risks of scabbing and scarring. It normally costs approximately

Quick Tip

About 50 to 75 percent of pregnant women get melasma, the "mask of pregnancy," which is caused by estrogen and made worse by exposure to the sun.

$500 per session and requires one to three sessions. (See Chapter 14 for more information about this procedure.)

Itchy Skin: Many women get itchy, dry skin in the latter stages of pregnancy. Although it won't prevent the drying out, moisturizing your face and body several times a day rehydrates your skin and should make you feel better.

Hair Care: Many doctors advise against dyeing your hair while you are pregnant, especially during the first few months. Many experts believe that high levels of exposure to the organic solvents used to chemically process hair can cause fetal harm. Yet, extensive studies on pregnant rats have shown no reproductive dangers from hair dyes, and no data exists at this time showing that dyes cause reproductive problems in humans. However, to be on the safe side, you may want to forgo coloring your hair your usual way. You can also try an alternative process that doesn't soak the scalp, such as highlighting done with a cap or with foils. You can also go for a vegetable dye that stains the hair without using chemicals. The only problem? You can't lighten hair color with vegetable dyes, only darken it.

Menopause: Staying Sane During the Change

Over the next decade, 10 baby boomers will turn 50 every minute, joining the growing ranks of the 76 million Americans approaching the half-century mark. According to the U.S. Census, one fourth of the country's population will be over 55 by the year 2000, but that is hardly making anyone slow down or succumb to the traditional stereotypes of aging.

Menopause brings many, many changes to a woman's body—some of which are very visible. The stage when ovaries shut down, reducing estrogen and progesterone levels, can come as soon as the early forties or take until your late fifties. Women going through menopause may suffer hot flashes, night sweats, vaginal dryness, insomnia, and rapid bone loss, all caused by the estrogen loss. Here are ways to counteract the symptoms of menopause:

Excessive Dryness: As you lose estrogen, you also lose some of the skin's natural moisture and need to find ways to add moisture back into the skin. The key here is to moisturize, moisturize, moisturize. The good news is that, because your skin produces less oil along with less estrogen, your acne breakouts may finally stop. You can also probably use oil-containing products without fear of breaking out. You can do a number of things in response to the changes in your skin's condition that can make it healthier and more glowing.

Use a mild cleanser to avoid further irritating your dry, sensitive skin. Alpha hydroxy products add moisture to the skin while stimulating the production of fresh collagen. An added boon: Alpha hydroxy acid products also help reverse sun damage.

Another choice you can make is to go on hormone replacement therapy (check first with your internist and gynecologist).

Dry Hair: As estrogen drops, your entire body gets drier, including your hair. Use mild shampoos and conditioners to treat brittle, dry hair as gently as possible. Avoid chemical treatments that can further weaken hair, such as straightening, using too hot a blow dryer, and perming your hair. If you color your hair, you may want to switch from permanent to semi-permanent dyes, which are less destructive to the hair shaft. The reason: semi-permanent dyes stain only the outside of the hair, while permanent dyes integrate into the hair's shaft, making it weaker.

Thinner Skin: The drop in estrogen hormone levels thins your skin. Before menopause sets in, the estrogen produced by your body causes your skin to be plumper, thicker, and moister. As estrogen levels fall with the onset of menopause, it causes your skin to get flakier and drier. As this happens, make sure to hydrate yourself from within by drinking lots of water. This will also help add moisture to parched skin.

Pasty Complexion: The blood vessels shrink down and get thinner with the loss of estrogen, so the skin looks slightly more sallow. Alpha hydroxy acid products and vitamin A preparations (such as Retin-A and Renova), as they stimulate your blood vessels, will bring back your pre-menopausal rosy glow. Exercise will boost your circulation, which will improve your complexion.

Brittle Bones: During menopause, bones become more brittle and muscles weaken. Fight back with calcium supplements and exercise. Not only will this increase your physical strength, it will also boost your metabolism.

Supplement Your Diet

These dietary supplements help combat hormonal havoc, whether you're suffering from PMS, dealing with a pregnancy, or coming to terms with "the change":

Vitamin B6: A daily dose of 50 milligrams (mg) of B6, combined with other B-complex vitamins, has shown some positive results, helping to reduce water retention, headaches, and breast swelling associated with hormonal fluctuations. Don't take any more than 100 mg a day, because larger doses provide no extra relief and can be toxic, causing numbness, tingling, and possibly nerve damage.

Vitamin C: When you feel sick or stressed, it's a good idea to take 500 to 1,000 mg per day of vitamin C.

Vitamin E: Like aspirin, vitamin E can inhibit the production of prostaglandins during the premenstrual period, which causes uterine walls to contract. To ease swelling and sensitivity, take 100 to 400 i.u. of vitamin E daily. Vitamin E supplements can also help alleviate dry skin.

Iron: Eat foods rich in iron, such as liver, broccoli, dried fruits and sunflower seeds, to help replace the iron lost through menstruation. Take a daily iron supplement of 15 mg.

Calcium: To avoid osteoporosis (brittle-bone disease) when you're older, doctors suggest 1,000 mg of calcium daily for women aged 19 to 50; women over 50 (menopausal) should ingest 1,500 mg of calcium daily.

The Life of Your Skin

We have discussed how hormones can affect your skin, both positively and negatively. Hormones change, not only with infrequent (although major) events like pregnancy, but ebb and flow through the years as you age, and affect the body and skin accordingly. Other factors, both internal and external, determine the health and appearance of our skin and body. Some things we can prevent (like how much sun exposure we get) and some we can't (like how much oil our skin produces), but at least what we can't prevent, we can usually do something about if we want to!

If you are interested in taking care of your appearance (and if you are reading this, you probably are), here is what you need to know about how your skin ages and what to do about it. If you take care of your skin from your twenties onward, your skin will stay in shape–just as your body does when you take good care of it.

So, here's to the life of your skin!

The Shape of Your Twenties

Your skin is in the best shape during these years of good production of collagen and elastin, which keep skin strong, firm, and flexible. The oil and moisture in your skin are well balanced, and you have excellent circulation throughout your body, including your skin. The skin on your face and body is, for the most part, smooth. Although you may tend to break out (especially around your menstrual cycle), and your skin may still be quite oily, it's not quite as bad as the pimples you got during the hormonally charged teen years. You may show tiny lines around your eyes, but most women in their twenties have skin that looks healthy and young. Despite the good state of your skin, you still need to watch out for beauty burglars, such as the sun, smoking, alcohol, and high-dosage birth control pills, which can cause adult acne breakouts, as opposed to lower-dose pills, which can actually help clear your complexion.

Your Skin Shape-Up Program
* Wash twice a day with an antibacterial cleanser if you are very oily. Otherwise, stick to a gentle cleanser.
* Zap any zits that pop up with 5 percent benzoyl peroxide.
* Use an alpha hydroxy acid product (such as glycolic acid) daily.

- Use an oil-free moisturizer with a minimum SPF of 15 (such as Purpose or Neutrogena).
- Use a higher SPF if you will be outdoors for anything more than 15 minutes. Start making sun protection a part of your life now and enjoy the healthy and beautiful results for the rest of your life.
- Start another lifelong habit: along with monthly breast self-exams, do a monthly skin check. Get familiar with your freckles and spots so you will be the first to notice if something changes or is new.

The Shape of Your Thirties

These years signal significant changes in your complexion. As you produce less oil, your skin becomes drier and scalier. Your nails may start to peel and crack as well. The accumulation of sun damage can begin to crop up in the form of fine wrinkles (especially in the crow's-feet area). Because your skin cell turnover is slower, you may begin to look slightly pasty, with less of a rosy glow. You may also start noticing age spots and other pigment discolorations. Your hair may start getting grayer and thinner; if thinning is severe, you might consider using Rogaine. You probably can't party the way you did in your twenties without sagging skin and dark circles under your eyes in the morning. Now, before you turn 35, is the time to start building bone mass to prevent osteoporosis, the brittle-bone disease. Increase any weight-bearing exercises you do (running, walking, working out with weights, jumping rope, etc.) and get enough calcium in your diet from dairy foods. Pregnancy may leave you with, among other things, spider veins and weight gain.

Your Skin Shape-Up Program

- Use a gentle cleanser to remove dirt without stripping your skin of moisture.
- Skip toners (they're too drying).
- Use a broad-spectrum UVA and UVB sunscreen *every day*.
- Start using a vitamin A derivative product to reduce sun damage and to speed cell turnover, and perhaps a vitamin C product. The antioxidants in vitamins A and C attack free radicals, which cause aging.
- Use a cream that contains alpha hydroxy acids daily and start a program of facial peels, either glycolic, fruit acid, or microdermabrasion, to help the skin stay toned and youthful.
- Take a good look in the mirror—it's probably time to start Botox for those fine lines and wrinkles forming around your eyes (see Chapter 9 for a complete description of this procedure).
- Take another step toward lifelong health and start visiting your dermatologist for yearly skin exams. Early detection of skin cancers and other problems is so important.

Did you know that...

Since 1975, the number of children born to women between 35 and 39 years old has increased by 43 percent.

The Shape of Your Forties

Your skin is getting drier and finer with the years, as sebum production slows down. This is good news if you've always had oily skin—now it's much less oily. By your forties you may notice increased lines and wrinkles on your face and hands. You may notice sagging at your jowls, neck, brows, and eyes due to loss of skin elasticity. Your hair is also getting lighter in pigment and shrinking in diameter, so it looks (and is) finer. The texture may also change. Some women even start to notice thinning at the temples by the time they turn 45. That postpregnancy fat and spider veins may still be around; in these and other ways you may think you're starting to look like your mother!

Your Skin Shape-Up Program

- Use moisturizing products and broad-spectrum sunscreens daily.
- Continue with alpha-hydroxy acid and vitamin A products (such as Retin-A).
- Avoid falling victim to the cosmetic counter salesperson's pitch for the latest "miracle in a jar." Your skin regimen doesn't have to be elaborate or even expensive to be effective.
- Liposuction of excess fat (on the neck, abdomen, legs, arms, almost anywhere) is a good option now; on the one hand, your metabolism is slowing, so you may not "burn off" those extra pounds on your own, but your skin still has good elasticity and will retract beautifully once the protruding fat is removed.
- Chemical peels and laser resurfacing can clear away many surface blemishes, blotches, and fine lines, and the skin still has good healing capabilities now.
- Consider Botox and/or collagen (or other filler substances) for facial lines and wrinkles if you haven't become a fan already.

The Shape of Your Fifties, Sixties, and Beyond

During these years your oil glands produce much less oil, less even than 10 years ago, making your entire body, face, and even scalp drier and flakier. You may start to notice more facial hair, especially around your chin and cheeks, which can be a reaction to the estrogen drop of menopause. You may start to suffer from hair loss. You may notice your body fat increasing as your metabolism slows down even further and you also need to eat fewer calories to maintain your present weight. If you are (and I hope you are) a healthy and active person, your appearance may start to bother you if you think you should look as young as you feel.

Your Skin Shape-Up Program

- Try using moisturizers that contain urea, lactic acid, and ammonium lactate to seal in moisture.
- Continue all the good habits that are hopefully second nature by now: daily use of sunscreen, alpha hydroxy acid, and vitamin A products and regular skin checks by yourself and your dermatologist.
- It's never too late to start facial treatments and Botox!
- Bleach facial hair or remove unwanted hair permanently with laser or electrolysis treatments.
- If you put off plastic surgery procedures before because you thought you were "too young," consider them now for areas that bother you, while you are young enough to enjoy the results! A blepharoplasty (eye job) is a relatively easy procedure with dramatic results, and of course a complete face-lift takes years off your appearance.
- Don't forget the basics—continue to eat a balanced diet and get enough exercise, rest, and regular medical screenings.

Myth:

You need a tummy tuck to get rid of excess fat after having children.

FACT:

Actually, liposuction will eliminate most "tummies" without any of the cutting, stitching, and anesthesia required with a traditional tummy tuck. Once the fat that protrudes from the area, creating the "tummy," is liposuctioned, the skin in the area will retract.

chapter eight

Diet Details

Life itself is the proper binge.
—Julia Child

HERE'S SOME FOOD FOR THOUGHT: SKIN IS THE LARGEST ORGAN OF YOUR BODY, occupying approximately 1.73 square meters to cover our flesh and bones. Since your body literally is your temple, you must treat it right by eating nutritionally, fortifying your skin with all the vitamins and nutrients it needs to stay healthy and glowing.

A balanced diet rich in complex carbohydrates (whole grains, fruits, vegetables), moderate in protein, and low in fat plays a role in how healthy you look and feel and in your energy level. Should you modify your diet to better suit oily, dry, combination, or even acne-prone skin? It may help some skin conditions, says Danielle Schupp, R.D., a registered dietitian and nutritionist at Reebok Sports Club in New York, New York, and in private practice. In this chapter she provides the latest information on eating to look your best and answers your most common questions about diet, nutrition, antioxidants, and even the BMI (body mass indicator).

Remember, if you have a family history of weight, high cholesterol, or other health problems, you should definitely consult with a doctor before planning a diet or food program.

General Rules for Good Nutrition

- Eat a balanced diet that includes a reasonable balance of carbohydrates, proteins, and fats.
- Make certain to consume at least five servings of fruits and vegetables a day.
- Drink at least eight, 8-ounce glasses of water a day.
- Include enough fiber in your diet, 25 to 35 grams per day.

Foods for Oily/Acne Skin

Aside from following the basic steps of sound nutrition, diet cannot significantly affect your skin if it's oily; in general, food that you eat will make your skin neither more nor less oily. Acne, however, can be affected by certain foods. If you find greasy foods affect your skin, try to limit those foods. Keeping a food journal may be helpful in determining which, if any, foods trigger breakouts.

Foods for Dry Skin

Dry skin may benefit from increasing fat in the diet. Women who are dieting to lose weight often cut out most of the fat from their diet. Eating a very low-fat or fat-free diet (with 10 percent or less of your calories coming from fat) can, over time, cause dry and flaky skin, which can make you look older. The lack of fat also usually makes your hair and nails brittle and weak.

I recommend that my clients keep a food journal to show what they are eating. Sometimes having it on paper is a good way to catch yourself in bad habits. It is also an excellent way to monitor whether you are eating enough fruits, vegetables, and fiber, and drinking enough water.

Here is an example of a menu of someone who is not eating properly and as a result may have dry skin. In the second menu, notice how I've added healthy fats back into the diet to nourish the skin.

VERY LOW-FAT MENU

Breakfast	Dry bagel and fruit salad
Lunch	Green salad with fat-free dressing and chicken
Snack	An apple and a dish of fat-free frozen yogurt
Dinner	1 bowl of pasta with fat-free marinara sauce and a side order of steamed veggies
Snack	One dish of fat-free frozen yogurt

IMPROVED MENU

Here, I've incorporated changes in the diet to increase fat.

Breakfast	1 slice whole grain toast with 1 tablespoon natural peanut butter, 1 glass of skim milk, a small banana
Lunch	Large green salad with 1 grilled chicken breast, 2 tablespoons oil-based (a vinaigrette type, not creamy) salad dressing, 1 small whole wheat roll
Snack	1 2-ounce portion of raisins and peanuts (a healthy way to incorporate fat)
Dinner	1 grilled salmon fillet (5 ounces), 1 small baked sweet potato, steamed spinach or broccoli
Snack	1 8-ounce bowl of low-fat or nonfat yogurt, ½ cup fruit salad

The Skinny on Fats

We need fats in our diet. Some fats are better for us than others. Fats made from plants (like avocado, nuts, seeds, and canola, sunflower, safflower, and soybean oils) lower total cholesterol and increase the good cholesterol (HDL). Fats from animal products (butter and the fat marbled throughout beef) and some plant sources (palm kernel and coconut oil), raise unhealthy cholesterol, which is a risk factor for cardiovascular disease. The best heart-healthy fats come from olives and nuts (like olive and peanut oils), soy (tofu), and omega-3 oils (oily fish); they lower unhealthy cholesterol, raise healthy cholesterol, and taste great.

HEALTHY FATS

MONOUNSATURATED	POLYUNSATURATED
Olives	Salmon (omega-3 oils)
Olive oil	Soybean oil
Canola oil	Cottonseed oil
Peanuts	Safflower oil
Peanut oil	Walnuts
Peanut butter	Mayonnaise
Avocado	

Note: Just because certain fats are healthier than others does not mean you can eat them in unlimited quantities! Eat these fats in moderation and choose them over unhealthy fats.

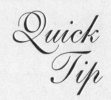

Quick Tip

Instead of dressing you can add a *few* pieces of avocado and small olives into a salad for an easy way to add healthy fat into your diet. Beware of adding too many, which can add a lot of calories to your salad.

Top 10 Foods for Overall Good Health

All of these foods can reduce the risk of getting cancer, diabetes, cardiovascular disease, and other chronic diseases:

Flax seed
Soy products (tofu)
Wheat germ
All deep orange and red-colored vegetables
Broccoli
Dark leafy green vegetables
Olive or canola oil
Fish rich in omega-3 oils (salmon, tuna)
Nuts/seeds
Avocado

Candy Is Not Dandy

Try to skip (or limit) fat-laden sweets like candy bars: the quick rush of energy they provide is followed by a blood-sugar crash that can leave you feeling even more tired. If you are looking for convenience, it's better to grab a nutrient bar–a protein or energy bar with about 16 grams of protein per serving. These bars give you more vitamins and minerals, plus carbohydrates, protein, and nutrients for energy, and they're low fat. However, they are a supplement, which means you still need to eat a good, balanced diet and shouldn't rely only on them to replace healthy foods. Another option: A medium-sized banana and a tablespoon of peanut butter.

Common Questions

Q: What types of vitamins should I take?

A: You should add a multivitamin with minerals (such as One-a-Day for women or men) to your daily diet, because, let's face it, most diets–even those that are well-balanced–may not provide all of the vitamins and minerals your body needs. For women, in particular, a multivitamin helps ensure that you're getting enough calcium, iron, and folic acid or folate (important for women planning to have children to prevent certain birth defects). Make sure the multivitamin you take has close to 100 percent of the daily value (RDA) of most vitamins and minerals. One thing to realize: unless you are deficient in a particular nutrient, megadosing on vitamins won't help to increase your energy or help relieve fatigue and may leave you with an upset stomach or, even worse, a toxic reaction.

Q: Well then, what kinds of supplements do I need?

A: Above and beyond the daily multivitamin, you may benefit from taking certain vitamins in higher levels to compensate for particular deficiencies:

Vitamin C (60 mg RDA): This vitamin is a very important antioxidant and 1,000 mg of vitamin C per day by mouth can help with sun damage or sun exposure. Because vitamin C is water-soluble, the body will excrete what it cannot use or absorb. The maximum amount of vitamin C an adult can absorb daily is 1,200 mg: achieving this usually requires 3 grams of oral intake of vitamin C (which is not recommended). If you are fighting off a cold or have a depressed immune system, you can take a vitamin C supplement of 500 to 1,000 mg per day.

Vitamin D (400 IU RDA): Vitamin D is also known as the "sunshine vitamin" because the body manufactures the vitamin after being exposed to sunlight. Ten to 15 minutes of sun exposure three times weekly is adequate to produce the body's requirement of vitamin D.

Vitamin E (30 IU RDA): Another important antioxidant, vitamin E–like vitamin A–is fat-soluble, so the body stores what it doesn't utilize. Vitamin E's antioxidant properties can help cardiovascular health by preventing cholesterol buildup in the artery walls. Vitamin E is also important for supple skin. Too much vitamin E can cause stomach upset and dizziness or even toxicity.

Thiamin (1.1 mg RDA): Thiamin helps enzymes metabolize carbohydrates and helps with nerve function. It is essential for normal development, growth, reproduction, physical performance, and well-being.

Pycnogenol: This powerful antioxidant can be found in certain vitamins.

Coenzyme Q-10: This enzyme also has potent antioxidant properties and is readily available as a supplement.

Riboflavin (1.3 mg RDA): This growth-promoting member of the vitamin B complex family facilitates metabolic reactions.

Niacin (15 mg RDA): Niacin, an essential vitamin in the body, helps to metabolize energy as well as to break down and synthesize fats.

B6 (1.6 mg RDA): This water-soluble vitamin helps in protein metabolism, neurotransmitter synthesis, and hemoglobin synthesis. Be careful not to overdose on your B vitamins. Studies show that greater than 100 mg of B6 may damage nerves in arms, legs, hands, and feet. Keep your dosage of B6 under 50 to 100 milligrams per day.

B-12 (2.0 mg RDA): This co-enzyme is necessary to metabolize fats; it also helps in nerve function and red blood cell formation.

Folate (200 mg RDA): This co-enzyme (also called folic acid) is involved in DNA synthesis and red blood cell formation. The RDA for women of child-bearing years is 400 mg to help prevent certain birth defects.

Q: What are antioxidants and why do I need them?

A: Antioxidants are compounds that can give your body a boost in deactivating harmful chemicals in the body known as free radicals. Free radicals are formed daily through normal body processes. They are also generated by environmental pollutants, such as cigarette smoke, automobile exhaust, and radiation. Free radicals are unstable compounds that can attack and injure vital cell structures. Certain vitamins

Quick Tip

It's a good idea to accumulate your sources of antioxidants from food rather than from supplements. The reason? You can get toxic doses of the vitamins over an extended period of time, especially vitamin E and selenium. In addition, foods contain other beneficial nutrients, providing a combined effect, whereas a supplement provides only the nutrient identified.

and minerals help our bodies to deactivate and minimize free-radical reactions within our cells. They also help with repairing the sun-related damage caused by free radicals and may also reduce the risk of skin cancers. These antioxidants are:

Beta Carotene: Found in orange and green fruits and vegetables (spinach, carrots, sweet potatoes, kale, apricots, and cantaloupe)

Vitamin C: Citrus fruits, broccoli, green and red peppers, and strawberries

Vitamin E: Vegetable oils, almonds, wheat germ, peanuts, sunflower and sesame seeds

Selenium: Seafood, meats, eggs, milk, whole grains, and garlic

Q: I've been hearing a lot about both green and black teas. What's the deal?

A: Both green and black teas have naturally occurring antioxidants. In recent studies, chemicals derived from green tea have stopped the growth of mouse skin cancers, reduced the incidence of lung cancer in mice exposed to tobacco carcinogens, lowered LDL (cholesterol) levels, and reduced blood clots in mice. In 1997, scientists at the University of Kansas found that green tea contains a possible cancer preventor, an antioxidant called epigallocatechin gallate. To boost health benefits, don't add milk to green tea: The antioxidant loses its potency when it binds with mild proteins. Take green tea capsules if you don't want the caffeine.

Q: What is the food guide pyramid and how can I use it?

A: The food guide pyramid is a general guide to daily food choices and is not an individualized diet for a specific person. It provides a general reference point regarding how many servings as well as the size of a serving for each food group the average individual may need per day. Here is a basic guide:

Starches/Grains	6 to 11 servings
Fruits	2 to 4 servings
Vegetables	3 to 5 servings
Protein	2 to 3 servings
Dairy	2 to 3 servings
Oils, sweets, alcohol	Use sparingly

Q: Can I eat a low-protein diet and still function well?

A: If your diet lacks protein, it is probably also deficient in zinc and iron, because animal protein is a good source for all three nutrients. By eating a diet with enough protein (65 mg per day, or 2 to 3 servings of 4 to 6 ounces), you'll help your body build and repair muscle tissue and body cells. By not eating enough protein, you can become malnourished, which can lead to illness, fatigue, and decreased concentration. Not sure about portion size? As a frame of reference, the size of a deck of cards is equivalent to about 3 ounces. Everyone needs certain amino acids, the building blocks of protein. If the diet doesn't provide these essential amino acids, over time the body breaks down its own muscle mass, with the consequences mentioned above. Deficient protein means deficient iron and zinc, which weakens the body and makes it more susceptible to illness.

Q: How can I increase iron in my diet?

A: You can get more iron in your diet by increasing your protein intake, eating iron-fortified foods, and taking a multivitamin. Many women need extra iron during their menstrual cycle, because when they bleed heavily they lose blood and therefore iron. Good sources of iron include: dark meats, seafood, milk and cheese, and iron-fortified cereals and breads. Plant sources of iron (iron-fortified cereals and breads, raisins, nuts, seeds, broccoli, prune juice) should be eaten with animal products or foods containing vitamin C to increase the iron's availability to your system. Drinking caffeinated coffee or tea interferes with iron absorption from these sources.

Q: What are the best foods for energy?

A: The best foods for increasing energy are complex carbohydrates: whole grain foods such as whole grain bread, bulgar, and oatmeal, brown rice, potatoes, and yams, fruits, and vegetables (which are less complex but still a good source for a quick boost of energy), as well as many vitamins and minerals. Unlike soda or candy, which result in a quick rush of sugar and then a crash, these carbohydrates (carbs) provide a good energy source and a bunch of nutrients.

Q: Do the new low-carbohydrate diets work?

A: Avoid low-carb diets. They are usually inadequate in complex carbs, vitamins, and minerals and ultimately will leave you feeling tired.

Quick Tip

Eating a little protein at each meal (i.e., a balanced meal as opposed to only a bowl of pasta) can increase production of brain chemicals that foster alertness. Any protein will help, but protein that is low in fat is healthier and will not leave you feeling as full and lethargic, because fat slows digestion. Try fish, skinless chicken, very lean beef, or low-fat yogurt.

Quick Tip

Are you drinking enough water? Check your urine. If it is dark yellow, this may be an indication that your body doesn't have enough water and is conserving it. If you are drinking enough water and eating enough fruit and vegetables (which are 75 to 95 percent water), urine will be clear and plentiful. Also, if you don't drink enough water, your skin won't be as supple or elastic as it can be and everything you eat is digested less efficiently.

When you lose weight from these diets, much of it is from water loss. Another problem with these types of diets is that most people can't sustain eating this way for a long period of time, so they end up gaining all the weight back

Q: How much fiber do I need?

A: You need fiber, because it's what helps to clean out your system. Generally 25 to 35 grams per day is recommended. Breads are a good source of fiber if you choose wisely; when shopping for a high-fiber bread, check the ingredient list. Avoid breads, that list "enriched wheat flour"–even though the label may say "high fiber," nutrients are stripped out and then "enriched" back in. To ensure that your bread is a good source of fiber, look for unprocessed whole grain products with 100 percent whole wheat or stone ground whole wheat on the ingredient list.

Q: What about the bloating I get when I eat fiber?

A: Many people go to extremes when it comes to fiber intake. They often take in very little fiber at first, and then start a high-fiber diet too quickly. Their systems simply haven't gotten a chance to get used to the added fiber, so they get bloated and gassy. The solution is to increase your fiber intake slowly. Also, most people don't realize that fiber doesn't work without water. Water pulls the fiber through your system, moving things along through the digestive system more easily and quickly and avoiding constipation. If you don't drink enough water, the fiber simply collects, loading down your system.

Q: How much water do I need to drink? I'm not a camel!

A: Relax. You don't need to drink until you can't hold anymore. Instead, follow this rule of thumb: If you are making more than one trip to the bathroom an hour, you're probably drinking too much for your body to handle, or for it to do your skin any good. Once your body is hydrated, no more moisture can get to your skin internally. When the body has become saturated, the kidneys, which are the prime filters of the blood and "balancers" of the body's water lever, will excrete any additional fluids that enter the body. Instead, you can further hydrate your skin by applying a topical moisturizer over damp skin.

Q: How does alcohol (the kind you drink) affect your skin?

A: If you drink alcoholic beverages in excess, it shows up in a sallow complexion, puffy face, and red eyes. Why? Because alcohol dehydrates your skin and causes blood vessels to dilate, creating puffiness under the eyelids and a generally puffy appearance. Drinking alcohol can also worsen a rosacea condition. Here are some of the other unattractive effects of alcohol:

A lowered resting muscle tone, which can make your face look drawn.

Because of its dilating effects, alcohol causes increased leakage of the blood vessels and capillaries, especially under the eyes, leading to puffiness of the lower eyelids.

Alcohol depresses the immune system, affecting the body's ability to fight off any low-level acne-type bacterial infections.

Alcohol also decreases absorption of several vitamins.

That's not to say nobody should ever have a drink. In fact, recent studies have suggested that drinking one glass of wine a day may reduce the risk of cardiovascular disease.

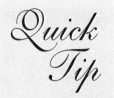

Quick Tip

It's a good idea to drink an extra cup of water for every alcoholic beverage you consume to help prevent dehydration (one of the causes of hangovers!).

Q: I've been hearing a lot about my BMI. What is it?

A: Both men and women can check their BMI (body mass index) to determine whether their weight is appropriate for their height (see BMI formula below). You can also use it to determine if you are seriously overweight and to estimate your risk of weight-related disease. The numbers are not foolproof. Some very muscular people may have a high BMI without health risks. Regardless of your BMI, if your waist is larger than 35 inches (if you're a woman, larger than 40 inches in a man), you have an increased risk of heart disease, diabetes, and other health problems.

BMI Formula

BMI = weight (pounds) divided by height (inches) squared and multiplied by 705.

Example: A 5'9" (69") woman weighing 145 pounds would do this formula as:

145 divided by 69 squared (4761) = .0304557, multiplied by 705 = 21.47

A BMI of 25 to 29 usually indicates a person is overweight (where risk to health begins); a BMI of 30 or more usually indicates a person is obese. The most desirable BMI is in the 19 to 24 range.

chapter nine

Reading Between the Lines

A loving person lives in a loving world. A hostile person lives in a hostile world. Everyone you meet is your mirror.
—KEN KEYS

THE LINES ON YOUR FACE REQUIRE SPECIAL HANDLING. HERE, WE'LL ANSWER common questions about how to deal with the most annoying ones.

Q: What can I do about the lines on my forehead?

A: The main reason you get forehead lines is from moving the frontalis muscle that stretches across the forehead. There is very little fat around this area, and the skin is very tightly anchored to the muscle, so gravity has very little effect on your forehead skin. What causes the wrinkling, then, is the contracting muscle. As the underlying muscle contracts, the skin covering the muscle pulls, causing it to pleat, like a curtain, and then to retract to its original position when the muscle relaxes. Over time, as the skin begins to lose its elasticity and becomes less elastic from sun damage, the constant contracting and relaxing of the muscle creates lines that eventually become etched into the skin. To the rescue: Botox injections, the best treatment for these kinds of lines.

Q: What about my crow's feet?

A: Just as with forehead lines, the underlying villain causing lines along the outer eye sockets (crow's-feet) is muscle contraction. To confirm this, simply look at yourself in the mirror and smile. As you smile, you'll notice the contraction of the areas where your crow's-feet are located; contraction is what causes wrinkles to form there. If that area doesn't contract when you smile, chances are you don't (and probably won't) have crow's-feet.

Any treatment that doesn't address the underlying muscle contraction won't produce good results. Again, your best bet here is Botox. Treatments take only a few seconds and the effect kicks in within several days. The results are terrific on two levels: first, you improve your crow's-feet in one fell swoop and second, you can then smile without closing your eyes.

When most people smile, their eye muscles contract until the eyelids practically cover their eyes. The Botox causes the muscles to stay relaxed during smiling, alleviating this problem. As with the forehead, some lines may be so deeply etched that relaxing the muscle doesn't completely solve the problem. In those cases, you can try laser resurfacing.

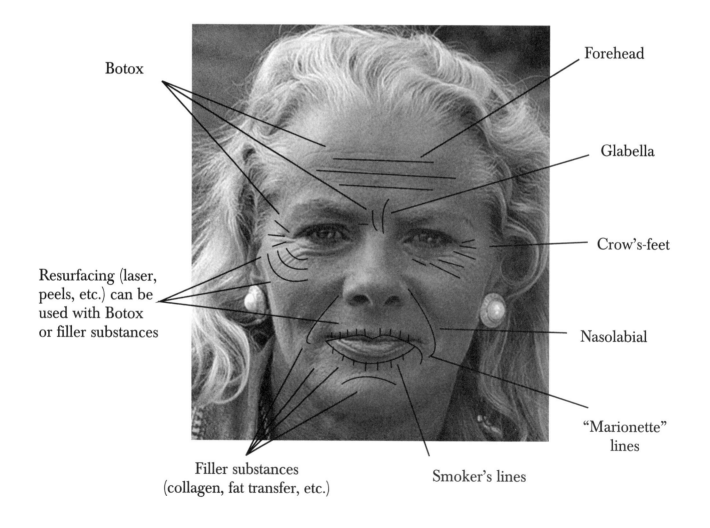

Botox

Forehead

Glabella

Crow's-feet

Resurfacing (laser, peels, etc.) can be used with Botox or filler substances

Nasolabial

"Marionette" lines

Filler substances (collagen, fat transfer, etc.)

Smoker's lines

What's Your Poison?

What It Is: Botox, the trade name for botulinum toxin, is a specific neuro-toxin that works wonderfully for getting rid of lines in the upper third of the face (particularly forehead creases and crow's-feet). Botox also works wonderfully for lines and wrinkles in the glabella (the area between the eyebrows).

How It Works: Botox works by interrupting the signal from the nerve to the muscle, so that when the brain sends its signal down the nerve, the muscle never gets the message. Botox takes about 10 seconds to inject and begins to take effect within a few days, gently relaxing the muscle, smoothing out the skin, and taking away the lines.

How Long It Lasts: Botox lasts from three to six months, the time it takes for the Botox protein to dissolve into the body. Because of the resultant "muscle retraining" effect of this protein, it seems that most people who continue to use Botox can go for a longer time in between treatments.

Strengths: People love how well it works at erasing the expression lines, and yet still are able to remain fully expressive when smiling, frowning, etc. Because it isn't an implant, no bulkiness ever appears beneath the skin.

Drawbacks: Botox doesn't work well for wrinkles on the lower part of the face (from the nose down).

Cost: The cost varies based on the amount of skin surface involved, which may encompass the crow's-feet, forehead, and glabella (the area between the eyebrows).

$500 for one area
$650 for two areas
$800 for three areas
$1,000 for four areas

Worst-Case Scenario

In some cases, lines may be so deeply etched into the forehead that even completely relaxing the muscles with Botox doesn't help. In that case, you can opt for laser resurfacing.

Botox is the perfect treatment for the upper third of the face, from the nose up. For the lower third of the face (from the nose down) you should go for a filler substance. The reason: the upper third of the face gets lines and wrinkles primarily from muscle action, whereas gravity and other environmental factors, rather than facial movement, do a number on the bottom third of the face.

Q: OK, then, what can I do for my lip lines?

A: Lip lines, also known as smoker's lines, appear along the outer lip border and the corners of the mouth. To treat lines around the lips, you must rely on either laser resurfacing or filler substances, or both.

Myth:

Botox injections can stop your heart.

FACT:

Botox is a purified derivative of botulinum toxin. When you eat food tainted with botulism, you can, indeed, become gravely ill. The form that dermatologists inject, however, has been used safely for years and stays just where it is injected. It is also so diluted that you'd have to actually drink many, many bottles of it for it to do any harm.

Quick Tip

You can combine autologous fat transfer with neck and jowl liposuction for fabulous results. In my practice, I refer to the combined procedure as the "weekend facelift." Patients who undergo fat transfer and/or neck liposuction on Friday are ready to return to work the following Monday, usually with virtually no discomfort and only occasional bruising or swelling, which are easily camouflaged with makeup.

Injecting a filler, such as collagen, into the lines offers a quick fix with no downtime. (Read on for more information about filler substances.) Fillers, unfortunately, tend to be rapidly absorbed into the high-movement areas around the mouth. Another option is laser resurfacing, which will correct the problem for the long term. Light chemical peels or microdermabrasion can also be helpful. I've found in my practice that the people who typically get collagen for their lip lines are models and other patients with high-profile careers with no opportunity for downtime. The rest go for laser resurfacing, taking into consideration that they'll need five to seven days of downtime, during which the skin is red and raw. (See Chapter 14 for more information about lasers.)

Q: The lines from my nose to the corners of my mouth are so deep and I'm starting to get them from the corners of my mouth down to my chin also.

A: The lines from your nose to your mouth (nasolabial folds) and from your mouth down to your chin (marionette lines) are primarily caused by shifts in gravity as the different triangular areas around both sides of the mouth move in opposite directions. The lower third of the face, from the nose down to the chin, tends to fall not so much from gravity as from the supporting tissue thinning and sinking directly toward the underlying muscle. Conversely, the cheek area and the facial area extending down to the jowls tend to fall slightly down and forward primarily from the force of gravity. This causes a shifting in opposite directions. Basically, when you're young, the triangular area around the mouth to the cheeks is in one even plane. As you age, the triangle around the mouth sinks inward, while the triangle comprising the cheek and jowl area moves in the opposite direction, out and down. There are several ways to try to correct this problem.

Fill 'er-Up

Filler substances comprise a group of materials designed to fill under the skin to plump up "lines" or "depressions." Fillers are especially useful for the area below the nose down to and around the chin.

Fillers also work wonderfully to fill in depressions left by acne and chicken pox scars.

If you are 35 or under and your skin is just beginning to thin, you can have your doctor inject one of the thinner filler substances, such as Collagen, Dermalogen, or any of the other collagen injectables, into the middle layer of the skin for a quick, easy fix. As you get beyond 35, collagen is frequently too thin to achieve the best results. Instead, you need to raise the entire area. This is best accomplished with a method called autologous fat transfer, or micro-lipo injection, a surgical procedure in which your own fat is removed and then put back into a line or wrinkle.

Autologous Fat Transfer

What It Is: This filler substance consists of fat taken from the patient's own body from a "donor site," usually the abdomen, hips, or buttocks. Because the fat comes from your own body, the risk of any type of allergic reaction is virtually nonexistent. The doctor usually withdraws more fat than is needed at the time and stores the extra fat for later use.

How It Works: A small amount of Novocaine-is injected into the donor site to numb the tissue. The fat is then gently suctioned into syringes and emulsified. Then the fat is injected into the recipient's facial area (usually the marionette lines or nasolabial folds, the chin area, or the area immediately below the lower lip). Because fat is a bulky substance, it works much better for deeper lines or defects than it does for thinner, more delicate lines.

How Long It Lasts: Although some of the fat will be reabsorbed into the body within six months, a portion of the transplanted fat will survive beyond that time. Many practices have found that by doing multiple, repetitive injections with the patient's own fat, results can last for as long as several years. In our practice, fat has proven to be extremely popular and extremely versatile, resulting in more dramatic and significant corrections than can be obtained with thinner substances, such as collagen.

Strengths:

* Fat is taken from the person's own body, so there is no way you can be allergic to it.
* Fat has a slightly longer staying period (especially if you get multiple injections).
* Because fat is bulkier, you can fill up deeper and larger defects. Fat transfer has also worked beautifully to plump up the backs of hands or even bony chest areas.
* Side effects are uncommon and usually consist of possible slight swelling or bruising.
* Once the fat has been obtained and stored for future use, subsequent injections of fat are quick and easy, taking about 10 to 15 minutes.

Drawback:

* You do need to take into consideration the fact that, because fat transfer is a two-part process, it is a more involved procedure than injecting collagen.

Cost: $1,500 for fat harvest and one initial injection to the face
  $2,000 for cheeks or hands
  $150 for each touch-up injection, using fat extracted from the initial procedure

---

Myth: Collagen in your skin care cream actually improves the collagen in your skin.

FACT:

Is collagen a cure-all? Not at all. True, it is one of the building blocks of healthy skin. However, applying collagen onto the skin gives no benefit whatsoever. Collagen is a very large molecule and thus completely incapable of penetrating through the skin. The large size of the collagen molecule is also why collagen treatments must be administered as in-office injections, the only way for the collagen to be delivered through the top layer of skin, the epidermis, into the deeper layer of skin where collagen resides, the dermis. So, don't spend extra money for anything that contains collagen in a cream.

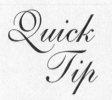

Collagen

What It Is: Collagen, which is derived from bovine, or cow, collagen, has been around for more than 20 years and is the most commonly used filler substance. The Collagen Corporation manufactures two injectable forms of collagen, Zyderm and Zyplast.

How It Works: The material is injected into the wrinkle or area you want plumped up (usually in the lower third of the face). This basic wash-and-wear procedure also holds an excellent track record for safety, effectiveness, and predictability.

How Long It Lasts: Collagen injections last for three to six months.

Strengths:

* Once you have been screened and cleared for collagen allergy, you can then proceed with collagen treatments.
* Collagen also allows the doctor a great deal of control and ability to inject exactly as much as he/she wants, precisely where it is needed.
* Collagen is formulated with a local anesthetic. To further reduce discomfort during the procedure, however, a topical numbing cream such as EMLA or Elamax 5 percent can be used.

Drawbacks:

* The main problem of collagen is that some people (about 3 percent of the population) develop an allergic reaction to it.
* It is not permanent. Collagen normally gets reabsorbed into the body over a period of three to six months, with lips and areas around the mouth reabsorbing faster than any other area.
* Because collagen is a thin substance and is injected into the dermis (the middle layer of the skin), you can inject only so much volume, limiting the degree to which lines and wrinkles in the skin can be corrected.
* The base molecule of standard, or bovine, collagen has been degraded to make it less allergenic. Unfortunately, this is part of the molecule that binds together the collagen compound, so after injection, collagen tends to dissipate faster than some other filler substances.

Cost: $400 per 1 cc syringe, which is enough to do either your lips or the nasolabial lines
$600 for 1½ cc syringes

Dermalogen

What It Is: Dermalogen is one of several offshoots of collagen currently available. It is extracted from human skin taken from a tissue bank; basically, it comes from the collagen of cadavers.

How It Works: In a method similar to organ transplantation, the collagen is screened, cleansed, and sterilized to remove any viral or infectious particles. Then the material is handled in the same way that hearts, livers, kidneys, and other donated organs and tissue are handled and prepared for transplantation.

How Long It Lasts: Three to six months.

Strengths:

- Because it comes from humans, the chance of an allergic reaction from this form of collagen is smaller than from bovine collagen.
- With human cadaver collagen, the connecting ends of the molecule are left intact, so it usually lasts longer than traditional collagen.

Drawbacks:

- For those people who are freaked out by using cadaver-donated collagen, it may not be worth the theoretical risks, which include contracting a viral infection such as HIV or hepatitis from human cadaver collagen.
- Unlike bovine collagen, Dermalogen was formulated without anesthetic (you can use topical numbing creams as discussed before).
- Despite some claims to the contrary, Dermalogen may not last any longer in the skin (three to six months) than bovine collagen.

Cost: $400 per syringe

Artecolle

What It Is: Artecolle is composed of micronized plastic beads and bovine collagen. This semipermanent filler is already in use in Europe and expected to come to the United States, pending FDA approval.

How It Works: After an injection, the collagen dissipates, leaving the plastic beads behind to plump up the skin.

How Long It Lasts: Reports from Europe claim that the beads stay put indefinitely.

Strength:

- The plastic beads last longer than collagen or Dermalogen, so the skin stays plumped up longer.

Drawback:

- Artecolle is not currently available in the U.S.

Cost: Not applicable at this time.

Hyaluronic Acid

What It Is: This filler is a natural and basic component of the human skin. Already in use in Europe, it is expected to be available in the United States within the next year, pending FDA approval.

How It Works: It's another component of the skin, like collagen, which can be injected to plump the skin.

How Long It Lasts: Four to six months.

Strength:

* It plumps up the skin with little or no potential for allergy.

Drawbacks:

* It is not FDA approved.
* Possible side effects include bumps and bubbles under the skin.
* Although it works well for deep lines, such as nasolabial folds, it does not work well for fine lines.

Cost: Not applicable at this time.

Autologen

What It Is: A form of collagen derived from the patient's own skin, typically after undergoing a large plastic surgery procedure such as a tummy tuck or face-lift, wherein a large amount of skin is extracted and sent to a lab and preserved (frozen) for later use.

How It Works: The patient's own collagen is extracted from her (or his) tissue, prepared, contained in sterile syringes, and sent back to the physician for injection.

How Long It Lasts: About three to four months.

Strength:

* Because you are using your own skin, there's no chance of an allergic reaction.

Drawback:

* Unless you are also undergoing a procedure that requires the removal of a large amount of tissue, this procedure can be impractical.

Cost: $2,000

Isologen

What It Is: Isologen comes from the person's own fibroblasts, the cells that produce collagen, which are extracted and sent to the lab to be harvested, cultured, and grown.

How It Works: A tiny "punch graft" of tissue is excised and sent off to a lab for processing; about eight weeks later (when it is first available) it's injected into the patient. Like seeds, the isologen is "planted" with the intention of "growing" more collagen in that spot.

How Long It Lasts: Requires several injections over a three- to six-month period. Because the fibroblasts are tiny, there is virtually no correction immediately evident. This procedure requires patience on the part of the patient, as it can take three to six months to see results. Then results can last one to two years.

Strength:

- Supposedly by increasing the number of fibroblasts in the area, the production of collagen in the area also increases.

Drawbacks:

- It takes about four months to see results between injections, which is not practical for some patients.
- Because this isn't a true filler substance that is injected with the purpose of immediately plumping up the area, there are no immediate results.

Cost: $500 per syringe

AlloDerm

What It Is: One of the newer fillers around, AlloDerm is an implant that is also culled from human cadaver tissue.

How It Works: Originally developed in 1992 for burn victims and reconstructive surgery patients, it is now used by many plastic surgeons as a cosmetic implant.

How Long It Lasts: Theoretically, forever.

Strength:

- The material is soft and pliable and can be folded, rolled, or stacked to fill out facial contours and larger areas of defect to be corrected.

Drawbacks:

- Because it is an implant, it doesn't work well on fine lines and wrinkles.
- If you decide to get a face-lift later on, you'll have to move the skin with the filler in it.

Cost: $2,000 to $3,000 per implant

Gore-Tex

What It Is: A thick, synthetic material made out of the same fabric used in winter outerwear that has been used in medicine for many years.

How It Works: In its standard form, Gore-Tex comes as individual threads, which are placed in the area in which you need elevation, such as the lips or nasolabial folds.

How Long It Lasts: Permanently.
Strengths:

* The material is inert (biologically inactive) so your body doesn't recognize it as something foreign, so allergy is extremely rare.
* It has an advantage over injectable fillers because it's permanent and won't get reabsorbed into the body over time like collagen and fat.
* If you don't like the result, the Gore-Tex can be removed.
* Requires only a local anesthesia.

Drawbacks:

* Gore-Tex presents some potential for some movement under the skin in the early stages (within the first six months after the procedure). If this occurs, the Gore-Tex may need to be removed and repositioned.
* There is a potential risk of infection, so a trained, skilled physician must insert the Gore-Tex under sterile conditions.
* It is slightly more expensive than some of the other filler substances.
* The recipient may experience a bit more swelling and bruising and, consequently, a little bit more downtime with the initial treatment of Gore-Tex than you'd find with fat or collagen.
* Many patients also dislike the fact that they can feel the Gore-Tex when they run their tongue along the inside of the mouth where the implant is.

Cost: $2,000 to $3,000, includes implant plus the surgeon's fee for lips and facial lines

SoftForm

What It Is: Another permanent implant, SoftForm is a version of Gore-Tex. It is sold by the Collagen Corporation.
How It Works: It comes in strips and is implanted into the skin.
How Long It Lasts: Permanently.
Strengths:

* It is great for filling up deep facial grooves and wrinkles.
* Requires only a local anesthetic, not general.

Drawbacks:

* Because the strips are linear, they don't quite fill all wrinkles, which tend to run in different directions.
* You may notice tiny stitch marks at the place of incision/implantation.
* The material needs to be placed exactly right, or you may see lines and bumps through the skin.
* As you move the mouth area, the implant may shift slightly.

Cost: $2,000 to $3,000, includes surgical fee and the implant, for lips and facial lines

chapter ten

Invest in Healthy Skin

Don't compromise yourself. You're all you've got.
–Janis Joplin

YOU CAN EASILY SPEND A FORTUNE AT THE DEPARTMENT STORE SEARCHING FOR JUST the perfect skin care cream–the one guaranteed to whisk away all your wrinkles with a touch of a finger. You'll also find no shortage of companies claiming (whether via television, print, or the Internet) that their products are the very ones you've been searching for. And let's not forget companies that invest heavily in fancy marketing and slick ads, all guaranteed to do one thing and one thing only– separate you from your wallet. With all that temptation out there, how can you be a savvy consumer? One way is to have your wits about you. It is a fallacy that you can find a miracle in a cream, lotion, or any kind of skin care potion. So, with the purpose of making your next shopping trip a little simpler (and perhaps cheaper), let's go through a rundown of which kinds of products you need, based on your budget (from $15 to $100) and your skin type.

I Have $15, What Should I Spend It On?

First, figure out whether your skin type is acne-prone, oily, combination, normal, or dry, and whether your skin is sun-damaged or sensitive. (See Chapter 1.)

Acne-Prone Skin

Here's my advice on what to do for acne-prone skin:
Start with a mild cleanser such as:

- Purpose Gentle Cleansing Wash, $5.99, 6 fl. oz.
- Basis Cleansing Bar (with astringents), $2.49, 4 fl. oz.

- Oilatum AD Liquid Cleanser $10.29, 8 fl. oz.
- PanOxyl 10% bar (10 percent benzoyl peroxide), $7.49, 4 oz.
- Neutrogena Oil-Free Acne Wash (salicylic acid), $6.49, 6 fl. oz.
- SalAc Wash (salicylic acid), $10.39, 6 fl. oz.

Add a 5 to 10 percent benzoyl peroxide preparation to be applied at bedtime (if you're not allergic), such as:

- Neutrogena Acne Mask (with clay and 5 percent benzoyl peroxide), $6.49, 2 oz.
- Clearasil 10 percent benzoyl peroxide, $4.79, .65 fl. oz.
- Persagel 10 (10 percent benzoyl peroxide), $4.99, 1 fl. oz.

Get an oil-free moisturizer with an SPF of 15 to use every morning, such as:

- Purpose Dual Treatment Moisture Lotion (oil-free, SPF 15), $9.99, 4 fl. oz.
- Neutrogena Moisture (oil-free, SPF 15), $11.79, 4 fl. oz.

Note

These are available with and without alpha hydroxy acids, which you may or may not want, depending upon how sensitive your skin is.

Many people who have acne also have a condition called seborrhea, which involves the oil glands of the face and of the scalp. To treat this condition, use anti-seborrheic shampoos at least twice a week for about eight weeks to reduce oiliness. Products include:

- T-Gel shampoo by Neutrogena, $5.13, 4.4 fl. oz.
- Head and Shoulders, $4.69, 15.2 fl. oz.
- Pentrax Shampoo, $14.49, 8 fl. oz.
- T-Sal shampoo by Neutrogena, which has salicylic acid as the active ingredient, $6.49, 4.5 fl. oz.
- Over-the-counter Nizoral AD Shampoo, $9.99, 4 fl. oz.

Oily Skin

Here's my advice on what to do for oily skin:

As I've mentioned before, many people with oily skin have an overlap with a condition called seborrhea, which involves the oil glands of the face and also the scalp. Use anti-seborrheic shampoos at least twice a week for about eight weeks to reduce oiliness. (See product list in preceding paragraph.)

Use a slightly drying cleanser, such as:

- Lever 2000 antibacterial soap, $1.99, two 5 oz. bars
- SalAc Wash, $10.39, 6 fl. oz.

Depending on how acne-prone you are, also use a 5 or 10 percent benzoyl peroxide cleanser or topical for nighttime to decrease oil output, such as:

- Clearasil 10 percent benzoyl peroxide, $4.79, .65 fl. oz.
- Persagel 10 (10 percent benzoyl peroxide), $4.99, 1 fl. oz.

At night, apply an ultra-light, oil-free moisturizer, such as Complex 15 Therapeutic Moisturizing Face Cream, $6.29, 2.5 fl. oz.

If you have extremely oil skin, you don't need additional moisture. Skip the moisturizer, and stick with a spray or gel sunscreen in the morning, such as:

- Neutrogena oil-free sunblock, SPF 30, $7.99, 4 fl. oz.
- Coppertone oil-free, waterproof, SPF 30, $9.99, 8 fl. oz.

Combination Skin

Here's my advice on what to do for combination skin:
Wash with a gentle cleanser, such as:

- Cetaphil Liquid Cleanser, $6.99, 8 fl. oz.
- Dove fragrance-free soap for sensitive skin, $2.69, two 4.25 oz. bars
- Purpose Gentle Cleansing Wash, $5.99, 6 fl. oz.

Then use an AHA- or retinol-containing product, such as:

- Purpose Alpha Hydroxy Moisture Lotion (oil-free, SPF 15), $11.99, 4 fl. oz.
- Neutrogena Healthy Skin Anti-Wrinkle Cream (retinol, SPF 15), $12.99, 4 fl. oz.

In the evening, cleanse with your morning cleanser and then use an AHA or retinol-containing moisturizer, such as:

- Pond's Age Defying Complex (oil-free, retinol, vitamins A and E, AHA), $10.99, 2 fl. oz.
- Basis All Night Face Cream (AHA, vitamins A, E, C), $7.99, 2 fl. oz.

Normal Skin

Here's what to do for normal skin:
Use a mild cleanser morning and evening such as:

- Cetaphil Liquid Cleanser, $6.99, 12 fl. oz.
- Fragrance-free Dove, $2.64, two 4.5 oz. bars

Moisturize and treat your skin with a product that has retinol and sunscreen, such as:

- Neutrogena Healthy Skin Anti-Wrinkle Cream twice a day–$12.99, 1.4 oz.

Myth:

If you have oily or dry skin, you are stuck with it for life.

FACT:

People who have oily skin in their youth may discover it gets drier as they age, especially after menopause in women. People who had acne in their teens can see it clear up as their hormones stabilize. People who never had a pimple before can develop acne in their forties. Hormones and environmental factors all affect how the skin behaves.

Dry Skin

Here's my advice on what to do for dry skin:

Start with a very mild cleanser, such as:

* Cetaphil Liquid Cleanser, which is about as mild as it gets, $6.99, 8 fl. oz.
* Neutrogena Extra Gentle Cleanser (fragrance-free), $7.69, 6.7 fl. oz.

Use an SPF-containing moisturizer for the morning. If you are not acne-prone, you can also use a product containing a few oils, such as:

* Eucerin Face Protective Moisture Lotion (SPF 25, fragrance-free), $8.79, 4 fl. oz.
* Neutrogena Intensified Day Moisture (SPF 15), $12.99, 2.25 fl. oz.
* Neutrogena Healthy Skin Anti-Wrinkle Cream (retinol, SPF 15), $13.99, 4 fl. oz.

For nighttime, use an alpha hydroxy acid–containing cream, with either glycolic or lactic acid, or a beta hydroxy acid, which will help your skin to exfoliate and also will act as a humectant, trapping and retaining water in the skin, such as:

* Oil of Olay Protective Renewal Lotion, Beta Hydroxy Complex (noncomedogenic), $9.99, 4 fl. oz.
* Pond's Age Defying Complex (oil-free, retinol, vitamins A and E, AHA), $10.99, 2 fl. oz.
* Alpha Hydrox AHA Facial Treatment (fragrance-free, oil-free, 10 percent glycolic acid), $10.99, 2 fl. oz.
* Basis All Night Face Cream (AHA, vitamins A, E, C), $7.99, 2 fl. oz.

Sun-Damaged Skin

This skin condition/type is characterized by increased pigmentation and freckling. Here's my advice:

Start with a mild cleanser, such as:

* Dove fragrance-free soap for sensitive skin, $2.69, two 4.25 oz. bars
* Cetaphil Liquid Cleanser, $6.99, 8 fl. oz.
* Purpose Gentle Cleansing Wash, $5.99, 6 fl. oz.

Use an SPF 15 or higher, oil-free moisturizer that contains either glycolic acid or another alpha hydroxy acid (such as lactic acid), or salicylic acid, a beta hydroxy acid, for example:

* Oil of Olay Protective Renewal Lotion, beta hydroxy complex (non-comedogenic), $9.99, 4 fl. oz.

- Purpose Alpha Hydroxy Moisture Lotion (oil-free, SPF 15), $11.99, 4 fl. oz.
- Alpha Hydrox AHA Facial Treatment (fragrance-free, oil-free, 10 percent glycolic), $10.99, 2 fl. oz.

For nighttime, use products from the vitamin A family (rather than vitamin C or E) that contain retinol to get the most bang for your buck, such as:

- Basis All Night Face Cream (AHA, vitamins A, E, C), $7.99, 2 fl. oz.
- Neutrogena Healthy Skin Anti-Wrinkle Cream (retinol, SPF 15), $12.99, 4 fl. oz.

Sensitive Skin

Here's my advice on what to do for sensitive skin:
Wash with a very gentle, fragrance-free cleanser, such as:

- Neutrogena Extra Gentle Cleanser (fragrance-free), $7.69, 6.7 fl. oz.
- Cetaphil Liquid Cleanser, $6.99, 8 fl. oz.
- Oilatum AD Liquid Cleanser, $10.29, 8 fl. oz.
- Dove fragrance-free soap for sensitive skin, $2.69, two 4.25 oz. bars
- Aveeno bar, $2.99, 3 oz.

Then, in the morning apply a light moisturizing product with SPF, such as:

- Oil of Olay Complete UV Protective Moisture Lotion (SPF 15, Vitamin E), $8.99, 4 fl. oz.
- Eucerin Face Protective Moisture Lotion (SPF 25, fragrance-free), $8.79, 4 fl. oz.
- Neutrogena Intensified Day Moisture (SPF 15), $12.99, 2.25 fl. oz.

In the evening, cleanse with your morning cleanser and then apply a moisturizer that contains a beta hydroxy acid (less irritating to sensitive skin than alpha hydroxy acids), such as:

- Oil of Olay Protective Renewal Lotion, Beta Hydroxy Complex (noncomedogenic), $9.99, 4 fl. oz.

I have $50, What Should I Spend It On?

Acne-Prone Skin

Use everything you would use in the $15 budget and add a glycolic acid product, such as NeoStrata FaceCream (15 percent AHA), $25, as a morning treatment, followed by an SPF 15 sunscreen, then makeup.

You can also add something in the vitamin A family, such as:

* Neutrogena Healthy Skin Anti-Wrinkle Cream (retinol, SPF 15), $12.99, 4 fl. oz.
* MD Forte Skin Rejuvenation Lotion, $25, 1 fl. oz.

If your skin is too dry, use an oil-free moisturizer, such as Hydrotone Lite moisturizer, $25, 2 fl. oz.

At nighttime, alternate back and forth between your vitamin A–containing product one night and your benzoyl peroxide–based product (from the $15 category) the next night.

Oily Skin

Use everything in the $15 budget, plus a vitamin A–containing treatment product at night to help curb excess oil, such as:

* Basis All Night Face Cream (AHA, vitamins A, E, C), $7.99, 2 fl. oz.
* MD Forte Skin Rejuvenation Lotion, $25, 1 fl. oz.

If you aren't allergic to sulfur, you can also try prescription sulfur-containing products. They work well on oily skin, because they dry and exfoliate skin and are also antibacterial/antiyeast.

Combination Skin

Use everything under the $15 budget, plus:

* GlyDerm Gentle Cleanser (contains glycolic acid), $20, 8 fl. oz.
* An AHA-containing sunscreen for the morning, such as NeoStrata Daytime Skin Smoothing Cream (with 8 percent glycolic acid and SPF 15), $25, applied in the morning after cleansing and before makeup

Normal Skin

Use everything in the $15 budget, plus:

* Cetaphil Liquid Cleanser $6,99, 8 fl. oz.
* GlyDerm Cleanser (2 percent glycolic acid cleanser), $20, 8 fl. oz.

In the morning use:

* Neostrata Daytime Skin Smoothing Cream with SPF, $25, 1.75 oz.

At nighttime use:

* Neutrogena Healthy Skin Anti-Wrinkle Cream, $12.99, 4 fl. oz.
* MD Forte Skin Rejuvenation Lotion I, $35, 2 fl. oz.

Dry/Sun-Damaged Skin

Dry-skinned people often have some form of sun damage, which disrupts the outer skin cell layer, preventing the skin from trapping and retaining water as well as it used to.

For $50, I would use everything in the $15 range with the addition of:

- An AHA-containing sunscreen for the morning, such as NeoStrata Daytime Skin Smoothing Cream (with 8 percent glycolic acid and SPF 15), $25, 1.75 oz., applied in the morning after cleansing and before makeup
- A vitamin A product at night, such as MD Forte Skin Rejuvenation Lotion, $25, 1 fl. oz.

Sensitive Skin

When you have truly sensitive skin, your itchy, inflamed skin rarely is a reaction to just a product or some other external factor on your skin. In fact, with sensitive skin, your skin often flares up in response to just about anything it comes into contact with as well as in response to foods you eat. As I've said before, the vast majority of people who may think they have sensitive skin don't have truly sensitive skin.

In terms of a routine for sensitive skin, it should not vary depending on how much money you have to spend. In this case, less is more. The fewer number of products and the fewer ingredients you can use, the better for this type of skin. All products should be fragrance-free, dye-free, and hypoallergenic.

Always cleanse with a mild, gentle cleanser, such as:

- Cetaphil Liquid Cleanser, $6.99, 8 fl. oz.
- Dove fragrance-free soap for sensitive skin, $2.69, two 4.25 oz. bars

Use as your moisturizer one of the following:

- Cetaphil Lotion, $10.49, 16 fl. oz.
- Cetaphil Cream for the body, $13.09, 16 oz.
- Purpose Dual Treatment Moisture Lotion (with SPF) for the face, $9.99, 4 fl. oz.

Use a sunscreen with a higher SPF, such as SkinCeuticals Ultimate UV Defense (SPF 30) or ROC Sunscreen (SPF 32), both of which are sold in doctor's offices for around $30.

I Have $100, What Should I Spend It On?

Acne-Prone Skin

Use everything in the $50 section, plus:

- A salicylic acid solution, like SalAc Wash, $10.39, 6 fl. oz.
- A morning cream with AHA and a sunscreen, such as NeoStrata Daytime Skin Smoothing Cream (with 8 percent glycolic acid and SPF 15), $25, 1.75 oz.
- A vitamin A–containing cream, such as MD Forte Skin Rejuvenation Lotion, $25, 1 fl. oz.

Stay with moisturizing products in the oil-free group, such as Hydrotone Lite moisturizer, $25, 2 oz.

Oily Skin

Follow the product guide for the $50 program, plus "play items" such as:

- Masks that contain benzoyl peroxide, glycolic acid, or mud. Masks can either hydrate, dry, or exfoliate the skin.
- Topical vitamin C patches for a quick fix.

Combination Skin

Follow the product guide for the $50 program, plus add a vitamin C product, such as:

- Citrix Cream, $70, 2 oz. (purchased through a dermatologist),
- Cellex-C, $75, 1 fl. oz.

Normal Skin

Follow the product guide for the $50 program, plus:

- Use either Cetaphil Liquid Cleanser, $6.99, 8 oz., GlyDerm Cleanser $20, 8 fl. oz., or Dove fragrance-free soap, $2.69, two 4.25 oz. bars
- In the morning use Neostrata Daytime Skin Smoothing cream with SPF, $25, 1.75 oz.
- At nighttime use Kinerase cream (a product containing botanical extracts purchased through a dermatologist) one night, $70, 1.4 oz., alternating the next night with MD Forte Skin Rejuvenation Lotion I (a vitamin A product that also contains vitamins C and E), $25, 1 fl. oz.
- Another option: Use Kinerase one night, and Citrix cream, $70, 2 oz., or Cellex-C, $70, 1 fl. oz., the next night.

Dry/Sun-Damaged Skin
Follow the product guide for the $50 program, plus:

* An AHA-containing sunscreen in the morning, such as NeoStrata Daytime Skin Smoothing Cream (with 8 percent glycolic acid and SPF 15), $25, 1.75 oz.
* A C topical, such as Citrix cream, $70 (purchased through a dermatologist), 2 oz., or Cellex-C, $75, 1 fl. oz.
* MD Forte Skin Rejuvenation Lotion, $25, 1 fl. oz.
* Lighten up brown spots or pigmentation with a product containing hydroquinone or kojic acid (applied either to the entire face or small areas), such as a lightening gel, $25, 2 fl. oz.
* Kinerase cream or lotion, $70, 1.4 oz..

Sensitive Skin
Follow the same program and product guide as for the $50 skin care budget.

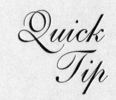

Quick Tip

When shopping at department-store counters, always ask for samples.

Shopping at a Pharmacy versus a Department Store

This is a matter of your own personal choice. There are good products, but no magic potion or remedy at the department store. In fact, if you're looking for "more bang for your buck," with the many wonderful prescription items now available, you would be better off scheduling a trip to your dermatologist for a consultation and a personalized routine involving the best of what the over-the-counter and prescription worlds have to offer. You can purchase numerous relatively inexpensive products at the pharmacy that will serve the same purpose and contain the same active ingredients as the more expensive items sold through department stores.

If a department store salesperson tries to get you to buy a glycolic acid or alpha hydroxy product, just ask what the product's pH factor is (how acidic it is) and what the concentration is. If you can't get a straight answer, it's better to nix buying the product, since you won't really know what you're getting.

Over-the-Counter Ingredients Checklist
Glycolic Acid Products (including AHAs): Require a pH factor of 3 or 4 with a concentration of from 8 percent to 20 percent.

Vitamin A (retinol) Products: Require a concentration of about 2 percent to 3 percent.

Topical Vitamin C Products: Require a low pH in the 2 to 3 range and a concentration of at least 10 percent.

INGREDIENT	POTENTIAL PROBLEM
ACNE-PRONE	
Mineral and other oils	Blocked pores; worsening of acne.
Petroleum jelly; petrolatum-containing products	Blocked pores.
PREGNANT OR NURSING	
Topical vitamin A family (retinol)	May cause birth defects.
SENSITIVE/ALLERGY-PRONE SKIN	
Fragrance	The leading cause of contact allergy from topically applied products.
Paraben/metylparaben preservatives	A small number of people are allergic to these.
Formaldehyde-type preservatives	Formaldehyde itself is seldom used today. However, Quaternium-15 is present in many topicals and can cause allergies. If you develop a persistent itchiness or irritation on the eyelids, it might be in your eye makeup. It can also lurk in nail polish and nail hardeners.
Acrylate group or Methacrylate	For people who have nail tips or wraps, this preservative can cause a contact dermatitis in and around the eye area from touching your eyes; you should avoid this preservative, especially if you experience any unexplained itchy or irritated skin on the face, especially the eyelids.
Active sunscreen agent, PABA (para-aminobenzoic acid)	About 1 to 5 percent of the population is allergic to PABA. If you are allergic to PABA, select a PABA-free sunscreen.
Propylene glycol	This preservative/stabilizer is present in many topical products and can cause sensitivity.
Alcohol	Can irritate skin. When it comes to makeup removers and eye makeup removers, many products may claim to be "alcohol free." However, they may substitute another solvent that, although technically not an alcohol, may be similarly irritating.

Ingredients Watch

Fortunately, most of the commercially available products in this country are responsibly produced, distributed, and manufactured. Depending on your skin type, you do need to be aware of a few areas. The chart on page 116 will help you determine which ingredients to steer clear of.

In general, if you have particularly sensitive or allergy-prone skin, you are best off looking for products that have relatively few ingredients. The greater the number of ingredients in a product, the more likely you are to develop an allergic reaction to something in the product or formulation.

Save Your Money

Cosmetics companies make a big deal about certain delivery systems, ingredients, and products that have nothing "big" about them except for their price. Here are some common industry buzz words to watch out for:

Liposomes: This is merely a type of delivery system, sort of like a delivery truck. So, the question to ask of anything touting liposomes is: what are they delivering? Certain companies would have you believe that having liposomes in their potions is something to get excited over, but it's like saying, "Aren't you excited that a delivery truck is pulling up to your house?" The answer is, not unless you know what is in the delivery truck.

Hyaluronic Acid: This large protein is present in the deeper layer of skin, but no scientific evidence exists that shows it is capable of penetrating into the skin when applied in a cream.

Epidermal Growth Factor (EGF): This protein helps stimulate the growth of epidermal cells (the top skin-cell layer). EGF has been shown to aid in the regrowth of skin in burn victims. However, it has not been scientifically proven to make a difference in healthy, normal skin.

Again, caveat emptor: let the buyer beware!

Shop Talk

To make sure you won't be taken for a ride, follow these savvy shopping tips before you shell out another cent:

- If you see a product you're interested in and it costs big bucks, ask the salesperson if you can try out a sample. Most salespeople will oblige, especially if it is a new product.
- Don't be taken in by a salesperson's fervent sales pitch that the product has worked for them, all their customers, and everyone else they can think of. Ask the salesperson to answer your specific questions, from what ingredients are in the product to how you need to apply it for best results. Go for realism over fantasy.
- When you choose an item that you've never used before, go for the smallest size you can find.

- Don't feel pressured by overeager salespeople (who mostly work on commission) to buy a product's entire line. That's why it's important to know your skin type. If you have dry skin, you most certainly do not need the toner.
- Remember: you shouldn't judge a cosmetic product by its package. Some of the best products are packaged inexpensively but deliver big results.

Common Questions

Q: What can I expect from a cosmetic product?

A: Flawless skin? Disappearing under-eye bags? No more wrinkles? Cosmetics companies in the grip of a marketing fervor often promise hope in a jar, pushing aside your realistic expectations of what a product can actually do, in favor of flights of fantasy. Unfortunately, that's just what these claims are–fantasy. Here's what you can really expect from quality topical products (both over-the-counter and by prescription): a slightly lighter and brighter complexion, plus minor improvement in very, very fine wrinkles. Any claims that go over and above these realities are simply that–unrealistic, unattainable claims.

Short of dramatic procedures, such as laser resurfacing or face-lifts, nothing out there will take twenty years off your looks. As the old saying goes, "If it sounds too good to be true, it probably is."

Q: What skin care products are on the FDA watch list?

A: At this time, the FDA continues to reserve judgment on the alpha hydroxy acids. The department is in somewhat of a quandary about this product area, because the FDA's current definition of a drug is anything with the potential to affect cellular structure. The FDA's job is to regulate drugs and foods, which by definition are those things that can affect the structure and function of an organ system. Any skin care product that does not affect structure and function is, by the FDA's definition, considered a cosmetic for over-the-counter sale. The problem is that the whole family of alpha hydroxy acids falls in between both definitions. This has created a new product classification called cosmeceuticals, a sort of hybrid between a cosmetic and a pharmaceutical agent or drug. In fact, the first available alpha hydroxy acid product, which was 12 percent lactic acid, is available only by prescription as a moisturizer called Lac-Hydrin lotion. On the other hand, a similar AHA called Am-Lactin, which is also 12 percent lactic acid, is now available over the counter.

This seeming duality is due, in part, to the changing environment. Alpha hydroxy products do seem to have some true biological effect on the structure and function of the skin. However, they appear to be so benign in most cases that, at least for the time being, the FDA has decided to steer clear of it, for fear of getting embroiled in a bureaucratic nightmare. But the jury is still out on this (metaphorically), and at some point, it is theoretically possible the FDA may step in and decide to regulate the alpha hydroxy acids.

Q: Do I really need that facial?

A: Patients ask me this question on a daily basis, and my answer is that, to me, facials (which involve cleansing, toning, exfoliating, extractions, masks, facial massage, and moisturizing) are similar to massages. They feel good, make you feel pampered, and that's nice. They can also help pop some zits that might be difficult for you to do yourself. However, they are no cure for a chronic acne or blackhead problem. If you get facials every month or so, and it's just a basic facial (no extra bells and whistles), I have no problem with that. What I do take issue with is when facialists or aestheticians tell you, "You're looking a little sallow today, let's add some oxygen to your facial"–and it's $25 more for the oxygen–or, "I have a wonderful collagen or marine extract treatment that will get rid of blood vessels"–and that adds another whopping $30 or $40 to your bill. I do have a problem with that.

Bottom line: facials really don't do anything medicinal long term for the skin (despite what some less-than-ethical salons claim). I also believe that if you end up in someone's hands who is inexperienced or unskilled, a facial poses some risk. In that case, the facialist may do harm by either overzealous pimple popping or extractions, which can lead to slight scarring, or by slathering the skin in heavy treatments, which can block pores. Personally, I have nothing against facials that are done properly, but you should know that what you are paying for is the experience and a temporarily more moisturized, smoother, and perhaps slightly tighter face.

My Favorite Products

I am frequently asked to list my favorite products. Sometimes patients ask me for products for a specific problem; other times I'm asked what my favorite products are in a given category.

Here is a selection of my favorite products for a wide variety of skin types and skin conditions, first by problem, second by category. All of these products are topical. If an "Rx" follows the product name, it means it is available only by prescription.

Acne

For use with all acne, including face, chest, and upper back.

Lever 2000 soap, for oily skin
Fragrance-free Dove, for sensitive skin
Benzac AC 2.5 percent wash, for normal skin (Rx)
Oilatum AD cleanser, for dry skin
Differin gel (Rx)
Avita cream (Rx)
Cleocin T pledgets, for oily skin (Rx)
Cleocin T gel, for normal skin (Rx)
Cleocin T lotion, for dry skin (Rx)
Triaz 6 percent gel, for normal skin (Rx)
Triaz 10 percent gel, for oily skin (Rx)
Novacet lotion (Rx)
Klaron (Rx)
Sulfacet-R, for overlapping acne/rosacea (Rx)
Azelex cream (Rx)
BenZac AC 2.5 percent gel, for normal to dry skin (Rx)
BenZac AC 5 percent gel, for normal skin (Rx)
BenZac AC 10 percent gel, for oily skin (Rx)
Head and Shoulders Intensive Treatment shampoo
T-Gel shampoo
Nizoral shampoo (Rx)
Purpose moisturizer

Combination Skin

Medicated shampoos: Nizoral (Rx), Head and Shoulders, T-Gel
NeoStrata Daytime Skin Smoothing Cream
Cetaphil or other gentle cleansers
Oil-free moisturizers
Avita cream (Rx)

Dry/Sensitive Skin

Fragrance-free Dove, for sensitive skin
Cetaphil Liquid cleanser
Oilatum AD cleanser
Cheer Free and All Free laundry detergent (fragrance- and dye-free)

Fragrance-free Curél lotion
Lubriderm lotion
Cetaphil cream and lotion
NeoStrata Daytime Skin Smoothing Cream (with 8 percent glycolic acid and SPF 15)
LacHydrin 12 percent lotion or cream (Rx)

Mature/Sun-Damage/Wrinkles

NeoStrata Daytime Skin Smoothing Cream (with 8 percent glycolic acid and SPF 15)
NeoStrata Face Cream (with 15 percent glycolic acid)
Avita .025 percent cream (Rx)
Kinerase cream
Lustra AF (with SPF 20 sunscreen), for lightening brown spots and pigmentation (Rx)
MD Forte Skin Rejuvenation Lotion I
Citrix cream (with 15 percent vitamin C)
Cellex-C
Azelex, for brown spots and pigmentation (Rx)
Cetaphil and other gentle non-soap cleansers
Hydrotone Lite moisturizer

Normal Skin

Fragrance-free Dove soap
NeoStrata Daytime Skin Smoothing Cream
Avita (Rx)
Differin (Rx)
Neutrogena Healthy Skin Anti-Wrinkle Cream
Citrix cream
Kinerase cream
Purpose Alpha Hydroxy Moisture Lotion with SPF

Oily Skin

GlyDerm Gentle Cleanser (contains glycolic acid)
Fragrance-free Dove, for sensitive skin
Vitamin A products: Avita (gel), Retin-A, Differin, Tazorac–(all Rx)
Sulfur products: Klaron, Novacet, Sulfacet–(all Rx)
Benzoyl peroxide products: Benzac, Triaz–(all Rx)
Clearasil Adult Care Tinted Cream
Clinac O. C. (Rx)

Rosacea/Seborrhea

Metrogel, for normal to oily skin (Rx)
Metrocream, for normal to dry skin (Rx)
Nizoral cream (Rx)
Klaron lotion (Rx)
Novacet lotion (Rx)
Sulfacet-R lotion (Rx)
Avita cream (may be too irritating for some; Rx)
Azelex (may be too irritating for some; Rx)
Clearasil Adult Care Tinted Cream (sulfer and resorcinol)
Head and Shoulders Intensive Treatment shampoo
Nizoral shampoo (Rx)
T-Gel and T-Sal shampoos by Neutrogena
Cetaphil Liquid cleanser
Oilatum AD antibacterial cleanser
Fragrance-free Dove, for sensitive skin
Purpose moisturizer (oil-free with SPF 15)

Here's a list of my favorite products by category:

Alpha Hydroxy Acids

NeoStrata Skin Smoothing Cream (8 percent glycolic acid)
NeoStrata Face Cream (15 percent glycolic acid)
NeoStrata Daytime Skin Smoothing Cream (8 percent glycolic acid, with SPF 15)
NeoStrata Body and Face lotion (15 percent glycolic acid)
Aqua Glycolic

Amino Fruit Acids

Excel (in-office treatments and at home products)

Benzoyl Peroxides

Benzac AC 2.5, 5, and 10 percent gels (Rx)
Triaz 6 and 10 percent gels (Rx)

Cleansers

Cetaphil Liquid
Oilatum AD
Fragrance-free Dove, for sensitive skin
GlyDerm Gentle cleanser (with glycolic acid)
MD Forte Facial cleanser II (with glycolic acid)
Lever 2000 antibacterial bar
Neutrogena

Purpose facial wash
Benzac AC cleanser (Rx)
Non-drying Antibacterial Cleansing Lotion by Topix

Hydroquinone (Lightening Agents)

Lustra AF (Rx)

Other Topicals (for rejuvenation)

Kinerase cream or lotion
Azelex (Rx)

Laundry Detergents

Cheer Free
All Free

Shampoos

Head and Shoulders Intensive Treatment
T-Gel
T-Sal
Nizoral (Rx)

Sunscreens

NeoStrata Daytime Skin Smoothing Cream
SolBar SPF 30 and 50
Purpose moisturizer, with SPF 15
Neutrogena moisturizer, with SPF 15
Total block SPF 60 by Fallene

Topical Antibacterial

Cleocin T lotion, gel, and pledgets (Rx)
Azelex (Rx)
Klaron (Rx)
Novacet (Rx)
Sulfacet R (Rx)
Metrogel/Metrocream (Rx)
Clearasil Adult Care Tinted Cream (sulfur and resorcinol)

Topical Anti-Yeast/Anti-Fungal

Nizoral cream (Rx)
Lamisil cream
Mentax cream (Rx)

Vitamin A:

Avita (Rx)
Differin (Rx)
MD Forte Skin Rejuvenation Lotion I
Tazorac (Rx)
Retin-A (Rx)

Vitamin C

Citrix cream
Cellex-C

More Favorite Products

I did a survey of the favorite skin-care products of the doctors and staff who work in the office at my center. Here is what they came up with.

Dr. Cynthia Gerardi (dermatologist):

* Aveda Shampure
* Avita Cream (Rx)
* Bobby Brown mascara, lipstick, pressed powder
* Citrix pads
* GlyDerm Body Lotion
* NeoStrata AHA Skin Smoothing Cream (with 8 percent glycolic acid)
* Z-cote sunscreen

Dr. Maritza Perez (dermatologist):

* Almay or Jacques DesSange mascara
* Christian Dior Dual Powder Foundation (made with cornstarch)
* Dermablend cover cream as a concealer
* Elizabeth Arden eye cream (with SPF 10)
* Elizabeth Arden lipsticks (with SPF 15)
* Jacques DesSange (Paris) eyeshadow
* Renova (Rx)
* Revlon Colorstay lipliner
* Roc SPF 32 physical sunblock
* SkinCeuticals SPF 30 hypoallergenic sunblock (physical and chemical block)
* SkinCeuticals Vitamin C Firming Cream

Products That Work from Women Who Work

These products are recommended by a group of women who work in my office at The Center for Dermatology, Cosmetic and Laser Surgery in Mount

Kisco, New York. The women polled include Dolores Croce, Lisa Feeney, Pam Ferraro, Janine Iodice, Katie Larson, Kathleen Raneri, and Ellen Starace.

- Almay Amazing Lash mascara (Janine, Lisa)
- Citrix cream (Lisa, Katie, Dolores, Kathy)
- Estée Lauder Double Wear Foundation (Janine)
- Eucerin Facial Moisturizing Lotion SPF 25 (Pam)
- Excel Cosmeceuticals cleanser (Pam, Lisa, Katie)
- L'Orêal Crayon Petite automatic lip liner (Pam, Dolores)
- MD Forte Skin Rejuvenation Lotion I by Allergan (Pam, Lisa, Ellen)
- Neostrata AHA Skin Smoothing Creme, with 8 percent glycolic acid (Katie, Dolores, Pam, Lisa, Ellen)
- Oil of Olay All Day Moisture Foundation (Kathy)
- Shiseido Rejuvenating moisturizer (Dolores)
- Ultima II eyeshadow base (Janine)

What Is In the Products You Buy?

Have you ever picked up a skin care or makeup product and looked, I mean really looked, at the ingredients? If you haven't, I suggest you start making it a practice. Despite their fancy-sounding names, some ingredients are quite simply generics, such as TEA Lauryl Sulfate for soap and Octyl Methoxycinnamate for sunscreen. Because it can be so confusing—and so important—I've asked Sheree Ladove, vice president of La Dove, Inc. and head of the La Dove Institute, a personal care research and development firm located in Miami, Florida, for her advice on the ingredients in products you use daily. Sheree is a leading cosmetic research and development formulator, with numerous celebrity clients, and she is an expert in natural cosmetic ingredient technology. Sheree's reputation for utilizing the world's finest ingredients has resulted in her being recognized and featured in more than a dozen national and international magazines. She is also a highly sought-after lecturer.

I gave Sheree some names of ingredients that you find in products in department stores, drugstores, retail chains, catalogs, and on the Internet. She helped to clarify each of them, backed up with research on the latest findings for each ingredient. I also asked her to tell us what she considers the best and worst ingredients for cleansers, masks, exfoliators, moisturizers, and so on.

Best Ingredients in Cleansing Products

Look for these ingredients in your cleansers (in addition to standard beauty boosters, such as alpha hydroxy acids, antioxidants, and vitamins):

Did you know that...

Graham Gordon Wulff, a South African chemist, invented Oil of Olay, which initially was used on British Royal Air Force pilots during World War II as a skin treatment to prevent dehydration of burn wounds.

Purified Water: Look for purified water as the first ingredient in the product. Water provides a fundamental source of pure hydration. It is non-irritating, noncomedogenic, and provides a clean base for good cleansing.

Propylene Glycol: Humectants that are oil-free, such as propylene glycol, help to hydrate without adding a greasy feel to skin.

Chamomile: Anti-irritants like chamomile are important in a cleanser. Chamomile was used by the ancient Egyptians for its healing qualities. It can help heal and soothe irritated skin.

Sodium Cocoyl Isothionate: This gentle cleansing agent, derived from coconut, is so mild it is frequently used in baby products.

Worst Cleansing Product Ingredients

Mineral Oil: This common component in wipe-off cleansers can clog pores and leave a greasy residue on skin. Another reason to shun mineral oil: it is very difficult to rinse off.

Ammonium-Based Surfactants: These are cleansing ingredients that are chemically reacted to create ammonium salts, such as ammonium lauryl sulfate and ammonium laureth sulfate. These can over-dry skin, leading to long-term irritation.

Soaps: These can dry and irritate skin and should be avoided, especially on sensitive skin.

Cocamide DEA, TEA Lauryl Sulfate, and Sodium C14-16 Olefin Sulfate: These detergent cleansers are known to be potentially serious skin irritants.

Best Mask Ingredients

A mask should help skin in one of two basic ways: it can be either a purifying (pure cleansing) treatment for oily/acne-prone skin or a hydrating/moisturizing treatment for dry, dehydrated skin. Whatever type of mask you choose, make sure it is formulated for your specific needs.

Kaolin: This is a pure Chinese clay that is great for oily skin and is used to gently extract excess oil from the skin.

Oatmeal: This common grain offers a soothing ingredient that helps eliminate irritation while it gently calms the skin.

Worst Mask Ingredients

Isopropyl Alcohol: Commonly known as rubbing alcohol, this ingredient can be severely drying to the skin.

Artificial Fragrance: Fragrances are believed to be responsible for the majority of all adverse reactions to cosmetics. Using a fragrance in a mask keeps this potential irritant on your skin for too long a duration and also poses the risk of fumes aggravating the eye area.

Peppermint, Menthol, and Eucalyptus: The potential for fumes to irritate the eye area makes these ingredients undesirable for facial masks.

Best Exfoliator Ingredients

AHAs: Alpha hydroxy acids loosen the glue between cells, helping them to exfoliate more rapidly.

BHAs: Beta hydroxy acids also loosen cells, gently increasing exfoliation. (AHAs and BHAs may irritate sensitive skin.)

Vitamin A: Helps to increase cell turnover, so skin exfoliates more quickly.

Jojoba: The exfoliating microspheres of jojoba (seeds) gently unclog pores and exfoliate dead cells. The jojoba microspheres are uniform in size and shape, which has been shown in clinical studies to be less irritating to the skin than irregularly shaped conventional exfoliants, such as apricot kernels, walnut shells, and pumice.

Papain: An enzyme found in papaya fruit, papain has a softening effect on tissues.

Worst Exfoliator Ingredients

Apricot Kernels, Walnut Shells, and Pumice: These ingredients contain irregularly shaped particles with sharp edges that can break capillaries in the delicate facial area.

Best Moisturizer Ingredients

Vegetal Squalane: This ingredient is naturally derived from olives and is enriched with a high percentage of lipids, a key component needed in moisturizers. Vegetal squalane has a high affinity to skin and is hypoallergenic.

Sodium Hyaluronate: Because of its high relative molecular mass, this ingredient actually fixes moisture on the surface of the skin and locks it in. It is an excellent water reservoir and an ideal lubricant.

Glycerin: This humectant helps to loosen dry skin scales and is extremely effective even on the most stubborn dry skin problems. A special bonus is that it does not aggravate acne.

Urea: Urea, like phospholipids, is a natural moisturizing factor that acts to attract and hold onto water at the skin surface. These particles work by binding water in place or by helping the skin rearrange its cellular proteins internally, which creates water retention. Urea is an effective moisturizer for dry skin and also has the bonus of not aggravating acne.

Vitamin C: Vitamin C helps promote the body's natural production of collagen, a vital element in maintaining the skin's firmness and elasticity. It also acts as a powerful antioxidant to fight against skin-damaging free radicals, which are stimulated by exposure to UV light, tobacco smoke, and other environmental hazards. It also improves the barrier function of the skin, helping the skin to retain moisture and reducing the appearance of wrinkles.

Worst Moisturizer Ingredients

Acetylated Lanolin: An ingredient derived from sheep's wool, acetylated lanolin is highly comedogenic and likely to cause skin to break out.

Cocoa Butter: Although it is an effective moisturizer, cocoa butter can irritate sensitive skin.

Fragrance: It is best to avoid fragrance in products. There is no good reason for a moisturizer to contain fragrances, because they add no moisturizing benefits and may be potentially allergenic or irritating.

Tallow: This ingredient is an animal fat that can clog pores.

PABA Sunscreen: Many people are allergic to PABA, an active ingredient in some sunscreens. It is potentially irritating and can sting. It causes allergies alone and in combination with sunlight. PABA also has a tendency to trigger acne.

Other Common Ingredients

Here are some ingredients commonly found in skin care products:

Jojoba Oil: Patches of jojoba are scattered throughout the Baja peninsula, south of California, the southern half of Arizona, and along the 1,000 miles of the western half of Mexico's mainland. Few plants can survive the temperatures, which reach 115°F, and the sparse rainfall (less than five inches per year in some areas) of these regions. Jojoba, however, has a built-in survival mechanism, because it needs no water during the summer when the rain almost never falls. During that time, the pores of the plant are completely sealed by a wax, thereby reducing the evaporation process that would shrivel any other plant. This unique coating is not only a moisture retention agent, but it also insulates the plant from the low nighttime temperatures of the desert. It translates to skin care by being an excellent moisturizer that can lay down a protective film, helping keep moisture locked into the skin.

Chamomile: Known to the Saxons as maythen, chamomile is one of the oldest-known English medicinal herbs. It was used by the ancient Egyptians for intermittent fevers. A number of species of chamomile grow in Europe, North Africa, and the temperate region of Asia. Four species can be found growing in England. Interest in chamomile has recently been revived, because of the discovery that it contains azulene. When isolated, this substance takes the form of blue crystals. It is said to be an excellent anti-inflammatory agent as well as an analgesic and an antiseptic. It is good for hypersensitive and dry skin, especially when there is redness or sensitivity.

Aloe Vera: Aloe vera has an ancient history. The use of aloe originated in Southern Africa. Aloe is a member of the lily family, but looks like a cactus. The inner chamber of the plant contains a clear gel-like pulp that contains "biogenic stimulators," which are used in skin therapy. The active ingredients of this pulp are organic acids, enzymes, amino acids, and polysaccharides. This makes aloe an excellent moisturizer. Chrysophanic acid, purported to be an important healing agent for the skin, has also been discovered in aloe vera gel. Legend has it that Cleopatra massaged fresh aloe gel into her skin every day to preserve her beauty.

Rosewater: The distillation of rose petals to produce rosewater almost certainly originated in ancient Persia. A document in the French National Library in Paris tells us that in A.D. 810, Persia's leading rosewater manufacturing province, Faristan, was compelled to provide an annual tax to the treasury of Baghdad totaling 30,000 bottles of rosewater. The art of distilling rose petals was introduced into the West by the Arabs during the tenth century; not long afterward, the French started to manufacture rosewater in the province of Avicenna. Rosewater is an especially mild moisturizer beneficial for all skin types, including the most sensitive.

Olives: The best-known cosmetic ingredient derived from olives is vegetal squalane. Vegetal squalane is produced by the hydrogenation of olives from Spain. Thanks to its perfectly defined molecular structure, its fixed and constant composition provides emollient and moisturizing properties.

Cyclomethicone: This silicone skin protector acts as a conditioning agent and has a good emollient feel.

Bisabolol: The soothing anti-inflammatory capacity of chamomile is delivered by one of its main components, bisabolol.

Green Tea: A green tea from Japan, polyphenols (catechins), acts as a powerful antioxidant. This potent free-radical scavenger is ten times stronger than vitamin E and 2.5 times stronger than vitamin C.

Camphor: Camphor is extracted from the bark of camphor trees. It was used as an early medicine for stimulating the clearing of nasal passages. Camphor is currently used in sports creams and acne medications, due to its drying effect.

Licorice: Recently researchers have discovered that licorice root offers excellent tyrosinase inhibition activity, making it the ideal natural ingredient to lighten skin, maintain an even skin tone, and reduce age-associated pigmentation changes.

Dead Sea Mud: What makes the Dead Sea so special is that its waters are very different from the waters of other seas and lakes. For starters, the Dead Sea has a higher concentration of salts (27 percent versus 3 percent in ordinary sea water). Second, the salt is of very different composition from the salt in ordinary sea water; the Dead Sea salts contain a small portion of sodium chloride (common salt) along with a high content of magnesium, potassium, and bromides. This special combination of minerals creates the perfect therapy for rheumatic conditions and skin disorders.

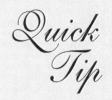

Quick Tip

Active ingredients in a product are those which orchestrate the product's performance. The product performance specifications dictate the level of active ingredients required. With regard to over-the-counter drug ingredients, the appropriate FDA monograph for specific drug ingredients dictates the level of actives required.

chapter eleven

The Acid Truth: Facial Peels

Action is the antidote to despair.
–JOAN BAEZ

I USE THE TERM FACIAL PEELS VERY CAUTIOUSLY. WHY? BECAUSE FOR TOO MANY of the folk who are 50 and older, the term facial or chemical peel conjures up images of men and women looking mummified and alabaster white, following doctors' stringent orders to avoid the sun for the rest of their lives, because they've basically had their faces burned off. While this scenario could, in some cases, apply to the deepest of all chemical peels–the phenol, or baker's peel–it has no relation whatsoever to many of the more popular, lighter peels, which are primarily made up of AHAs.

Separating the Peels
Today's AHA peels couldn't be any more different from phenol peels in their effects, benefits, and downtime. To make the benefits and effects of each abundantly clear, so nobody gets confused, I'll separate the peels into those that are deep, medium, and superficial (light).

Deep Peels
The Buzz: These are phenol-based peels. Phenol is the name of a very caustic chemical that burns the skin. These deep peels are highly effective but extremely powerful, which means they must be done with extreme caution and by a physician with a significant amount of experience with doing this kind of peel. Although they can work well on very deep lines, deep peels pose some danger, because you can't control the chemical once it starts burning its way into the skin. You usually

131

are under general anesthesia during these peels, and the downtime is significant—two weeks.

Another huge downside: your skin turns pure white after the peel, and then you need to stay out of the sun for the rest of your life. In my opinion, these kinds of peels are a little too extreme for almost any skin problem. If your lines are really deep, I recommend laser resurfacing, which is a much more controllable procedure. These peels are useful for extremely severely sun-damaged skin and very deep wrinkles, such as around the mouth.

Active Ingredient: Phenol, a caustic chemical.

Treatment Times: One in-office treatment under general anesthesia. Effects are essentially permanent.

Recovery Downtime: At least two weeks.

Cost: $3,000 to $5,000.

At-Home Routine: Sun must be avoided forever after. Home care usually involves use of sunscreen, an alpha hydroxy cream, and Retin-A.

Medium-Depth Peels

The Buzz: These highly popular peels depend on an active ingredient called TCA, or trichloracetic acid. They are performed in the office, with or without anesthesia.

These medium-depth peels:

Work wonderfully for sun damage and pigmentation discoloration;

Give slight improvement of fine lines and wrinkles;

Have a minimal effect on acne scars;

Have no effect on sagging or hanging skin (which needs laser resurfacing; see Chapter 14).

Active Ingredient: TCA (trichloracetic acid).

Treatment Times: One in-office treatment, which lasts for two to five years.

Recovery Downtime: Five to seven days.

Cost: $1,500 for full face; $1,500 for hands; $1,500 for chest.

At-Home Routine: Your regular home maintenance program, which may include sunscreen, alpha hydroxy acids, and vitamin A and C derivatives.

Superficial (Light) Peels

The Buzz: During lighter, or aptly named lunchtime peels, men and women literally come in during their lunch hour, receive a facial treatment, and immediately after return to work. Superficial peels are the most popular and most commonly performed group of "chemical peels."

They normally consist of either alpha or beta hydroxy acids and a mixture of anti-irritants that exfoliate skin on a deeper level (far better than at-home exfoliants and gels). They also unclog pores, stimulate collagen production, and smooth out the skin's surface, reducing fine lines and wrinkles. One significant advantage is that they are far less irritating to the skin than any other chemical peel process.

The most common ingredient used in superficial peels is glycolic acid, a member of the alpha hydroxy acid group. The alpha hydroxy acids are a group of naturally occurring compounds. Glycolic acid, which is derived from sugar cane, has the smallest molecular structure of the alpha hydroxy acids, which allows it to more easily and effectively penetrate the skin. You can get a low-concentration (20 to 30 percent) glycolic acid facial treatment or peel in either the doctor's office or in spas or salons. In higher concentrations (50 to 70 percent), you need to go to a physician. Even at higher concentrations, though, glycolic acid is a very mild peeling agent, and in no way gives the final result of deeper peels or laser resurfacing.

These superficial peels:

Work wonderfully for fading pigmented areas, including freckles and melasma. With repetitive treatments of glycolic acid peeling (exfoliation), the skin will develop a smoother, brighter, and clearer complexion;

Give slight improvement over fine lines and wrinkles;

Have a minimal effect on acne scars;

Have no effect on sagging or hanging skin (which needs laser resurfacing; see Chapter 14).

Active Ingredient: Glycolic acid or a similar alpha hydroxy acid/anti-irritant compound.

Treatment Times: A series of up to six treatments, performed as frequently as once a week or as infrequently as once a month, depending on the intensity of the peel and on the patient's schedule.

Recovery Downtime: None.

Cost: $125 per alpha hydroxy–based peel (also $125 per beta hydroxy peel).

At-Home Routine: To obtain the best result with glycolic facial treatments, most patients need to simultaneously follow an appropriate home routine. This routine usually includes a product containing glycolic acid, sometimes a topical vitamin A product as well, and perhaps even a vitamin C–containing product.

A Shopping Guide to Superficial Facial Peels

It's a popular concept: Run to the doctor during your lunchtime and get a peel. The upside: There is no downtime (read, recovery period), and you can return to work looking healthy and glowing. Which superficial peel is best for you? Here's the scoop on finding the peel with the most appeal.

Glycolic Acid

What It Is: Glycolic acid is the most common of all the alpha hydroxy acids. Manufacturers usually combine it with anti-irritating ingredients in a mild formula for home use.

Benefits: Glycolic acid peels give you a smoother, brighter, and clearer complexion by sloughing off dead skin cells, and they reverse the process of photo-aging by increasing the production of collagen by fibroblast cells. The peels also help erase fine lines and wrinkles.

How It Works: Glycolic acid peels exfoliate the top layer of your skin while simultaneously eliminating dead skin cells and excess oils that can clog pores. Within a few weeks of regularly using glycolic acid products, your skin should begin to appear smoother and healthier. Fine lines seem to disappear, and your complexion appears more even. Glycolic acid peels may cause mild tingling when first applied, but the sensation is rarely uncomfortable, depending on how sensitive your skin is. As the dead-cell layer sloughs off, your skin may appear slightly drier than normal. Once the new, smoother-looking skin comes in, your complexion will appear more youthful and vibrant.

Treatment: Most people undergo a series of six weekly treatments, building up the concentration and contact time with each peel. Products can be used twice daily, once in the morning and once in the evening, unless your physician directs you otherwise. Glycolic acid products can be used with other moisturizers and cleansers. However, if you have oily or acne-prone skin, make sure your other facial products are noncomedogenic and non-irritating.

Where: Glycolic acid is mainly used for in-office peels and in at-home products. In-office concentrations 20 percent to 70 percent; at-home 8 percent to 15 percent.

Cost: $125 per peel (also $125 for beta hydroxy peels).

Downtime: None.

The Softer Side of Peels

Amino Fruit Acids

What It Is: Amino fruit acid peels are the next generation of power exfoliators, developed in response to the skin sensitivity and irritation experienced by some glycolic acid users. They are made up of the amino acids found in the seeds and buds of sugar cane.

Benefits: As with glycolic acid peels, these peels improve skin tone, normalize skin cells, and boost collagen production. On a personal note, in my practice we've had significant experience and great results with the amino fruit acid peels. Many patients who have been unable to tolerate glycolic acid in higher strengths have tolerated the amino fruit acid peels quite well and have received very nice results.

How It Works: The amino acids found in the seeds and buds of sugar cane are refined through certain chemical reactions and converted into acids, which supposedly have an antioxidant effect (neutralize free radicals) and increase the skin's moisture retention. These acid peels differ from glycolics in that they are chemically buffered by amino molecules, which makes them less irritating. The addition of vitamin C also boosts their effectiveness.

Treatment Times: Most people receive a series of six weekly treatments, building up concentration and contact time with each facial.

Where: In the office.

Cost: $125.

Downtime: None.

Refinity

What It Is: This peel was developed by Collagen Corporation to reduce the irritation associated with AHA products. Basically this is a 70 percent glycolic acid solution that contains an anti-irritant, strontium nitrate, which Collagen calls Cosmaderm 7. Studies show that concentrations of 20 to 30 percent of strontium nitrate are shown to significantly reduce irritation.

Benefits: The same as with glycolic acid peels and amino fruit acid peels.

How It Works: Because Refinity contains the anti-irritant ingredient strontium nitrate, it allows people with sensitive skin to tolerate higher concentrations of glycolic acid without the associated irritation. Otherwise, it has the same effect as other glycolic acid facials.

Treatment Times: Six treatments once a week or every other week.

Where: Available in many physicians' offices.

Cost: $125.

Downtime: None.

Laser Facials

What It Is: Currently, the only true "laser facial" is one offered through the Soft Light Thermolase system. It is a combination of a very delicate Neodymium YAG laser along with its proprietary carbon-based lotion. A "laser facial" is not the same thing as laser resurfacing.

Benefits: Same as with glycolic acid facials, amino fruit acid peels, and Refinity.

How It Works: The laser gives a mild exfoliation, which is comparable to glycolic acid facials. But because these facials take about 45 minutes to perform, as opposed to the five minutes it takes to do a glycolic acid peel, it's not worth it. Usually, these facial peels also cost a lot more than glycolic acid peels

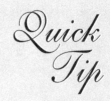

Quick Tip

I usually suggest having a glycolic acid facial to patients looking for a way to brighten up their complexion. But some people, especially those with sensitive skin, can experience skin irritation from the formulation. In those cases, I suggest trying either the less irritating amino fruit acid or Refinity facial.

and their counterparts, which doesn't make them very cost effective. In my opinion, they offer nothing over glycolic acid, amino fruit acids, or Refinity, and that's why I seldom recommend them to patients.

Treatment Times: Approximately 45 minutes; six treatments, every one to two weeks.

Where: Doctor's office or spa.

Cost: Mild facial, $140; peel, $195.

Downtime: None.

The Next Step: Power Peels (Microdermabrasion)

If patients have several skin problems they'd like to correct that a regular peel, such as glycolic acid, amino fruit acid, or Refinity (which are mainly used to freshen up the complexion), isn't strong enough to handle, I suggest they go to the next step in treatment: power peels, a.k.a. microdermabrasion and Dermapeel.

What It Is: Introduced in Europe a few years ago, microdermabrasion, or a power peel, is a fast, painless choice for clearing up minor skin problems. These peels use tiny aluminum oxide crystals to achieve the result. The other peels (besides laser) use chemicals or liquids.

Benefits: A series of treatments can improve the appearance of acne scars, fine wrinkling, sun-damaged skin, and pigmentation problems, such as melasma, dark spots, and freckling. This process provides a viable option for those who don't have time for laser resurfacing.

How It Works: First, a machine is used to spray the skin (face, neck, hands, thighs, buttocks) with aluminum oxide crystals, which are extremely fine—smaller than grains of sand. The crystals are then vacuumed up through another chamber of the hand-held machine, in the process exfoliating the skin's outermost layer, leaving the skin baby soft, with a healthy glow. As the tiny particles go whizzing by, they cause a very, very fine sanding and polishing effect.

Treatment Times: Like all lunchtime treatments, a power peel requires a series of treatments—usually six—to get maximum results. The treatments can be performed as frequently as once a week or as infrequently as every three to four weeks. As with glycolic acid–type peels, you usually need to apply topical alpha hydroxy preparations or vitamin A products at home simultaneously to get the best results.

Where: Physician's office.

Cost: $175.

Downtime: None.

Unlike traditional dermabrasion, which requires anesthesia and in which the outer layer of skin is completely removed, microdermabrasion causes no pain or scarring. In fact, when the treatment is complete, the skin is smooth and soft with a pink glow. The patient can immediately return to work, as opposed to dermabrasion, which requires one to two weeks for the patient to recover. The analogy that I use is that microdermabrasion is to dermabrasion what a hand grenade is to a nuclear bomb.

The Powerful Advantage of Microdermabrasion

This treatment, in my experience, offers several potential advantages over the other mild lunchtime chemical peel treatments. In my opinion, microdermabrasion is more effective in getting rid of fine lines and wrinkles, at reducing brown spots, freckle-type pigmentation and age spots, and especially at refining mature or sun-damaged skin. If you have blocked pores and blackheads, the combination of the small exfoliating crystals and the action of the machine's vacuum is great for the skin. It may also offer a slight advantage in reducing mild acne or chicken pox scars. It offers some mild benefits against fine wrinkling in the crow's-feet area. If any of these skin conditions is an issue with one of our patients, we frequently recommend microdermabrasion. Otherwise, the liquid glycolic treatments are just as effective as microdermabrasion.

Alphabet Soup

I usually have my patients do some sort of regular at-home skin care routine, just as a dentist recommends regularly brushing and flossing your teeth. That routine often includes vitamin A, vitamin C, or alpha hydroxy cream. For more substantial improvements, patients can get their skin glowing via a glycolic acid facial, amino acid facial, or Refinity. If they have any particular skin problems to deal with, they undergo microdermabrasion. If their skin really needs a lot of work, I recommend laser resurfacing.

I call this alphabet soup, because the vitamins A and C make up a wide spectrum of topical preparations that you can apply to your face as at-home treatments.

Vitamin A

What It Is: The vitamin A family is probably the most important in terms of improving the appearance of your skin.

Researchers discovered 15 years ago—when Retin-A, a derivative of vitamin A, was originally designed as an acne product—that it enhanced people's complexions and reduced fine lines and wrinkles.

The active ingredient in Retin-A, tretinoin, is the only chemical to receive FDA approval for anti-aging and anti-sun-damage purposes.

Because the original formulation of Retin-A was designed for acne users, many adults found it too drying and too irritating. Now several other topical vitamin A derivatives are sold both by prescription and over the counter (such as retinol and retinyl palmitate).

Here are a few vitamin A–based prescription products:

Retin-A Micro: A recent prescription preparation from Johnson & Johnson, the same company that makes Retin-A, Retin-A Micro uses microsphere technology (a time-release formula that releases the tretinoin overnight), which allows for a more sustained use over time. Although it is less irritating than the original Retin-A, many adults still find the Retin-A Micro to be somewhat drying or irritating.

Renova: This product is also from Johnson & Johnson, and like Retin-A and Retin-A Micro, it also has tretinoin as its active ingredient. The difference here is that the tretinoin is delivered in a mineral oil–based moisturizing cream. The only downside is that some patients develop acne cysts from the mineral oil in Renova. If you are not acne-prone, this is a wonderful preparation.

Avita: Avita is available in both a cream and a gel by prescription. Avita has been our most popular formulation of tretinoin for adults, who use it for complexion smoothing and wrinkle reduction, because it doesn't irritate skin and doesn't contain the potentially pore-blocking mineral oil found in Renova.

Differin Gel: This prescription treatment is made up of a molecule called adapalene, which makes it less sun-sensitizing than tretinoin, so it's great to use on kids or when you're out in the sun. It works well on acne and also helps make your complexion glow. Differin is not as effective as preparations containing tretinoin for making a complexion look better when it comes to improving pigmentation problems, such as melasma or freckles.

Tazorac: This prescription product is the newest member of the group. The active ingredient is tazarotene. It's extremely dry and irritating. If you have particularly oily skin, it can help acne as well as stubborn blackheads on the nose. But it is not particularly useful for adults with dry or sensitive skin, and it is too harsh for the average female patient.

As for the over-the-counter A-team members: Both retinol and retinyl palmitate are two over-the-counter vitamin A active ingredients, and can be found in products by Lancôme, Elizabeth Arden, Eucerin, and Neutrogena. As long as the product contains at least 3 percent of a vitamin A derivative, that is enough for it to be effective–but not as effective as a prescription vitamin A product. However, if you have sensitive skin, even the small amounts in these products can irritate your skin.

Take Your Vitamin C

When applied in a topical preparation to the face, vitamin C can help reduce free radicals, which lead to skin-cell damage, which increases the risk of getting skin cancer. But don't think that if you apply it to your face, vitamin C will help produce collagen or stimulate fresh collagen to get rid of wrinkles. Its main function is to fight against further sun damage, not to actively restore the skin itself. Consider it as more like a security guard than a contractor.

For maximum effectiveness, topical vitamin C needs to meet several requirements:

- The concentration must be at least 10 percent of the vitamin C active ingredient. This is key to the effectiveness of the product. Don't go any lower, or the product loses its effectiveness.
- It needs to have a relatively low pH in the range of 2 or 3.
- It must be packaged in a fairly opaque bottle and stored in a dark place, because any exposure to sunlight will cause it to break down and stop working. For example, if the bottle is left sitting on the window sill, it will go from 10 percent active to only 1 percent active.
- Vitamin C is also rather unstable and may have an increased risk of becoming inactivated or breaking down when applied with other topical agents. Therefore, in our practice we recommend that patients apply vitamin C by itself or with a sunscreen or moisturizer, but preferably not with a topical vitamin A or alpha hydroxy acid.

Potent C

There are several ways to take your vitamin C. Here is a rundown of vitamin C product options:

Serums: These are slightly thinner and less moisturizing than creams. Supposedly, the solution is stable, but the products do tend to lose their potency and turn brown in a few months. Products to try: Cellex-C, SkinCeutical's Serum.

Patches: These deliver doses of vitamin C directly into your skin, without exposing it to air, which degrades or dilutes it. You wear the patches at home (similar to the smoker's patch). Products to try: University Medical Facelift Vitamin C Antiwrinkle Patch, Sudden Change Line and Wrinkle Patches (one type with antioxidant vitamins C, E, and A, and one type with alpha hydroxy acid patches).

Creams: The dosages vary from one cream to another. Products to try: Citrix cream, University Medical Facelift Cell Regeneration Cream (10 percent vitamin C).

Capsules: These seal in the vitamin C in lotion form, minimizing the opportunity for it to degrade. Product to try: Avon's Anew Formula C-Facial Treatment Capsules.

Quick Tip

If you've worried about developing sun sensitivity after using a tretinoin-based product, such as Renova or Retin-A, you can relax. It has been recently discovered that after three months of continuous usage of any of the tretinoin-containing products, sun sensitivity is dramatically reduced.

Other Vitamins

Vitamin E: Americans have an ongoing love affair with topical vitamin E. Never has so much noise been made about a vitamin with so little science behind it. Here's what's known: Vitamin E acts as an antioxidant, meaning it protects skin from damage by free radicals. When it is taken by mouth, it can have a whole host of potentially beneficial effects. Applied to the skin, however, no evidence exists to support any benefit at all. We tell our patients that if a topical product contains vitamin E and is the same price as the next product, then go for it. But we don't recommend spending extra money for a product simply because it contains vitamin E.

Vitamin K: Here is another vitamin that has had a tremendous amount of misrepresentation. When taken orally, vitamin K helps the body with its clotting systems. When applied topically, it may help lessen bruising as a by-product of helping to improve the clotting of superficial blood vessels. However, I want to make the point that absolutely no effect of vitamin K on broken blood vessels or capillaries has been documented; broken blood vessels are simply intact blood vessels and have nothing to do with clotting.

Lunch Menu

Here are some quick ways to get skin glowing during your lunch hour:

* Get a glycolic acid, amino fruit acid, or Refinity peel.
* Get a power peel (microdermabrasion), which polishes skin in 20 minutes, and you can see the difference after one or two treatments.
* Get saline injections to get rid of spider veins as well as Botox injections to reduce any deep furrows or crow's-feet—to help you look wide eyed and refreshed. (Botox should be injected only in lines that are caused by muscle action, in the upper third of the face.)
* Get collagen injections to plump up the lines on the lower part of your face and on and around your lips.
* Get an endermologie treatment to help reduce cellulite (see Chapter 17).

Common Questions

Q: Should I get my facial treatment (peel) in a salon or a doctor's office?

A: Many of these treatments are available at both the salon and the doctor's office. Some of this is determined by state law, which differs from state to state. Individual practitioners also might opt to provide some treatments but not others. When the decision is yours to make, you need to weigh several variables.

First, most responsible spas or salon owners allow only licensed cosmetologists/aestheticians to perform very, very mild-strength chemical peels or microdermabrasion, which is the correct policy. If you're looking for a very mild treatment for less money than you'd have to spend if a physician was doing your peel, then it makes sense for you to get your treatment at either a spa or a salon. You do need to keep in mind two potential problems: If a complication occurs (some type of irritation, infection, early scarring, or pigmentation problem) is the spa or salon equipped to handle it or do they have a dermatologist with whom they deal directly? If so, will you be charged for any visits to the doctor, or does the spa or salon plan on taking care of the bill?

The advantage of getting the procedures done in a physician's office is obviously that the practicing physician is capable of and equipped to handle any complications that may arise.

Because a spa or a salon will give you a far weaker concentration (read, watered-down version) of the active ingredient, whether it's glycolic acid or vitamin C acid, than you would get from a dermatologist, you might want to consider whether it is worth the money.

I would probably consider receiving a peel at a spa or a salon if it is part of a facial and you enjoy the pampering. But if it means paying considerably more money, beyond the typical charge for a facial ($75), then you should have the treatment done by a physician.

Q: What are AHAs and how do they work?

A: AHAs are alpha hydroxy acids, a family of naturally occurring compounds that have several properties in common. All AHAs cause increased exfoliation of the outer layer of skin, and unplug pores. They also function as a humectant to moisturize, or hydrate, the skin, because they tend to help trap and pull water into the skin. In addition, with regular use they can help reverse sun damage in the top layer of skin (the epidermis) while stimulating or causing some fresh collagen and elastin to grow in the deeper layer of skin (the dermis). AHAs are wonderful substances from nature that can help treat everything from acne to dry skin, sun damage, and general complexion enhancement.

Q: I breathe oxygen for free, why do I need to pay for it in a facial?

A: My feeling is that these facials are a lot of hot air. They are often touted by spas and salons as delivering a blast of 100 percent pure oxygen to your face after an exfoliation and a basic facial with an oxygen cream mask. Proponents claim that these facials boost cell metabolism, making the skin look younger by ridding it of nasty wastes and toxins. Here's why they don't work: Oxygen from the atmosphere is readily available to our tissues by breathing through the lungs, from which oxygen is carried by our red blood cells to our skin in a usable form.

So, unless you have an open wound you are trying to drive oxygen into, because it can't get there through the body's normal circulation as in a diabetic foot ulcer, added oxygen, whether in the form of products or a facial, delivers no benefits to healthy, normal skin, because oxygen cannot enter through healthy, intact skin.

However, oxygen *can* work to rejuvenate the skin through a treatment administered in a hyperbaric oxygen chamber. In this situation, oxygen at high pressure is inhaled through the lungs, helping to bring more oxygen to the blood. This "hyper-oxygenated" blood then delivers improved oxygen levels to all of the body, including the muscles, internal organs, and the skin, helping skin to look younger. The effects of a hyperbaric oxygen chamber can beat back the effects of beauty burglars (stress, lack of sleep, smoking, and sun damage), all of which contribute to decreased blood flow to the skin, causing a sallow complexion and a dull skin tone.

An added bonus: An oxygen treatment can help alleviate headaches, stress, and anxiety, and it is great if used after an operation or cosmetic surgery procedure to speed healing.

chapter twelve

Let the Sun Shine

Keep your face to the sunshine and
you cannot see the shadow.
—HELEN KELLER

I'VE SAID IT BEFORE, AND I'LL SAY IT AGAIN: "THERE IS NO SUCH THING AS A healthy tan." Please, let this be your mantra too. A tan is your body's direct response to ultraviolet light and to skin injury. It is the skin struggling very hard to protect itself against any further damage—not a pretty picture. The greatest cause of skin damage and premature wrinkling is being caught unprotected during incidental sun exposure (like walking to your car, driving in your car, checking your mail outside, walking your dog, or sitting by a window). Many women spend their teenage and early adult years soaking up as much of the sun as possible. Later, they seem to suffer the consequences of their idle youth, when they notice age spots, dark patches, rough textures, broken blood vessels, and other results of sun exposure. They come to me seeking help, crying about their "lost beauty." Skin that doesn't glow with health can be devastating to a woman's self-esteem.

Sun exposure damages skin in many ways. First, it attacks the epidermis, the thin outermost layer of skin. Then, it damages the upper layers of the dermis, or the bulk of the skin, leaving them thinner, less resilient, and more susceptible to wrinkling. Over time, the collagen and elastin fibers that form the dermis also break down, causing gradual drooping and sagging.

In this chapter, I'll give you ways to protect yourself, the right way to apply sunscreen, products to use that protect against both UVA and UVB rays, plus the newest (most natural) ingredients thought to help prevent skin cancer.

A Prescription for Sun Damage

When women come to me suffering from sun damage, I give them the facts, and the news is sobering. According to the American Skin Cancer Foundation, about a million cases of skin cancer are diagnosed in the United States each year, and it is striking at increasingly younger ages, often before the age of 39. Clearly, these numbers show that every time you go out in the sun, you are virtually taking your life in your hands—that is, unless you are taking the proper measures necessary to protect your skin. What are these measures?

According to the American Academy of Dermatology, everyone should use a broad-spectrum sunscreen having an SPF of at least 15 and containing ingredients that screen both ultraviolet B (UVB) and ultraviolet A (UVA) rays. Ingredients that screen UVA include benzophenone, titanium dioxide, zinc oxide, butyl methoxydibenzoylmethane, Parsol 1789.

Stop Focusing on Tanning

I tell my patients to forget about focusing on getting a tan and to start focusing on preventing sun damage by using sunblock or sunscreen. I tell them they should assume they will naturally get some sun almost every day. In fact, most people don't realize that sun damage from UVA and UVB rays doesn't happen only while sunning at the beach. You can also get sun damage from incidental exposure, which is, just as it says, incidental. Incidental exposure occurs every time skin that is unprotected by sunscreen comes in contact with the sun's rays. It occurs when you're in your car driving and the sun gets to you through the closed window. It occurs on cloudy days, when you haven't put anything on to protect your face. It occurs when you are out on the slopes, skiing. The effects are cumulative and can result in sun damage and eventually even skin cancer.

Skin Cancers

The sun can change the nature of melanocyte cells (the cells that cause the skin to tan), making them abnormal and in rare cases malignant. Because this process occurs over a period of 10 to 20 years, the damage doesn't show immediately. Diagnoses of skin cancer have doubled annually since 1980, according to the American Cancer Society. The Skin Cancer Foundation reports that women who rarely use sunscreens have been found to have twice the melanoma risk of women who virtually always use them. Women who reported that they tanned moderately after burning and never used sunscreens were the most vulnerable group, with approximately four times the melanoma risk as those with the same skin type who used sunscreens.

There are three forms of skin cancer:

- Basal cell: This is a non-melanoma form of skin cancer. According to *The Lancet* journal, about 1.2 million cases of basal-cell carcinoma were diagnosed in the U.S. in 1998, and the incidence of skin cancer in parts of Europe has more than tripled during the last 14 years.

  The most common type of basal-cell skin cancer tends to show up on your face or other sun-exposed areas. Since the growth is usually small and red, it is often mistaken for a persistent zit. The cancer rarely spreads to internal organs, but if it is left unchecked for many years (around 10), it could eat away at your skin.

- Squamous cell: This non-melanoma form of skin cancer can kill. Between 1980 and 1989, the incidence of non-melanoma skin cancers increased by 65 percent. Squamous-cell cancers also show up in sun-exposed areas, but usually take the form of slightly scaly or hard patches that won't heal. These cancers pose a greater potential to spread internally than do basal-cell cancers.

- Melanoma: This is the least common, but the deadliest, of the skin cancers, causing nearly 10,000 U.S. deaths per year (one American dies every hour of melanoma). Between 1980 and 1989, the incidence of melanoma in the U.S. increased by 21 percent. By the year 2000, as many as one in 75 Americans may develop melanoma at some time during their lifetime. However, melanoma is not automatically a death sentence. With early detection and early removal, it can be completely cured.

  Melanoma is usually a dark or multicolored growth that, unlike basal- and squamous-cell cancers, which occur most prevalently on the face, can begin anywhere on the body. It is more commonly seen on the trunk: For men, the upper back is the most common area on the body; for women, the lower leg, bottom of the feet, or calves is more common. Melanoma also is tied more closely than are the non-melanoma cancers to intermittent intense sun exposure. So, for example, sustaining a single bad sunburn in childhood or taking a once-a-year vacation to a sunny place can increase the risk of melanoma. Conversely, chronic sun exposure and cumulative sun exposure—for example, a farmer who is chronically exposed to sunlight while working in the fields—are the primary causes of basal- and squamous-cell cancers.

  Melanoma is striking at increasingly younger ages; 25 percent of the more than 30,000 people expected to develop melanoma this year will be 39 or younger.

Myth:

You're not at risk for skin cancer if you're rarely out in the sun.

FACT:

Regardless of your sun-exposure habits today, you probably had more than enough sun exposure during your childhood to put you at risk for skin cancer. Not only that, but just running your daily errands can give you enough sun exposure to increase the possibility of skin cancer.

The incidence of skin cancer may further increase, if, as some scientists predict, the earth's ozone layer continues to deplete. According to the Environmental Protection Agency, scientists began accumulating evidence in the 1980s that the ozone layer—a thin shield in the stratosphere that protects life on earth from UV radiation—is being exhausted through the use of certain chemicals at a rate of 4 to 6 percent each decade. This means that increasingly more UV radiation is reaching the earth and our skin, and affecting our bodies.

Sun-Care Glossary

Here are some definitions of terms to help you better understand the language of sun protection.

Antioxidant: The fire extinguisher that diffuses, puts out, or takes the energy hit from free radicals (see below), sparing and protecting the surrounding skin cells from damaging free radicals. Some antioxidants are vitamins A, C, and E.

Free Radicals: When the skin is exposed to ultraviolet light, it forms high-energy molecules called free radicals, which cause damage to neighboring skin cells as these radical molecules discharge energy. Antioxidants can render the molecules harmless. By using products with antioxidants, you can help diminish any further harm to your skin.

SPF (Sun Protection Factor): SPFs range from 2 to 60. The number refers to the sunscreen's ability to block out the sun's harmful rays. The SPF amount indicates how much longer you can stay in the sun before getting a sunburn while wearing the sunscreen than you could without the protection. For example, if your unprotected skin normally burns in 10 minutes and you wear an SPF of 15, you are protected about 15 times longer, or for 150 minutes. Keep in mind that your skin's burning time changes depending upon the strength of the sun each day.

Sunscreens: Sunscreens get into the skin and sit there like a line of defensemen. When ultraviolet rays hit the skin, the sunscreen grabs them and absorbs the dangerous energy before it gets into the skin cells.

Sunblocks: These sunscreen products block the ultraviolet light, causing it to reflect off the skin, so it never gets into the skin in the first place. Think of it as having a mirror sitting on the skin's surface.

UVB Rays: Short-wave, intense ultraviolet light that radiates from the sun. UVB rays penetrate the skin, causing it to show a visible burn, which is the first warning sign you are getting too much sun. Most older sunscreens on the market protect only against UVB rays.

UVA Rays: Long-wave, intense ultraviolet rays that can deeply penetrate the skin, even through windows and loose-knit clothing. UVA rays cause sun damage (dryness, wrinkling, discoloration) to the skin and affect the production of collagen and elastin, which give skin its structure and firmness. Unlike the burn you get from UVB rays, the effects of UVA sun damage are not immediately apparent. Failure to block UVA accounts for why the dark spots on many women's faces get worse, especially when they use a high SPF sunscreen, because the SPF blocks only the UVB.

UVC Rays: You don't need to worry about the effects of UVC rays on your skin: these ultraviolet rays of sunlight never make it to earth; the ozone layer blocks them.

An Early Problem

In the early days, we knew much more about the UVB rays than we did about UVA. The UVB rays of sunlight are much hotter and more intense than UVA rays, and older sunscreens absorbed only these rays. The problem arose when people started applying sunscreens to prevent sunburns and ended up staying out in the sun longer than they ever could before. The result? More UVA damage and an increased incidence of skin cancer. Once researchers realized what was happening, they began formulating second-generation, broad-spectrum sunscreens that help block both UVA and UVB rays.

What Are the Best Sunscreens?

Many excellent products in various formulations are available for you to choose from. What's wonderful about these products is that they block not only the short-wavelength, ultraviolet B light of the sun but also the longer-wavelength, ultraviolet A rays.

Sunblocks

Some sunscreens contain a finely milled total blocking agent, such as zinc oxide or titanium dioxide, which is sometimes called Z-Cote on labels. The older versions of these products looked opaque white. The newer products have only a tiny hint of a white hue, because the particles are so finely ground. The particles are absorbed by the skin, fending off even more of the sun's rays. Both micronized ingredients are especially good for sensitive, freckle-prone skin, because they're natural and don't cause the rashes that sunscreens with PABA can. In addition, the newer Parsol 1789, also known as avobenzone, is a very good sunscreening agent, although it is not a total block like zinc oxide or titanium dioxide. Avobenzone does provide good broad-spectrum protection, however, because it screens both UVA and UVB rays.

Here are some good sunscreen products:

Ombrelle SPF 15 and 30
Neutrogena UVA/UVB sunblock, SPF 15, 30, and 45
Coppertone Shade UVA Guard SPF 30
Coppertone Waterproof Sunblock
BioSun Oil-Free Gel

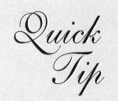

Quick Tip

Your eye measures only visible light— where most of the light comes from the sun's direct beam. UV light, however, is invisible to the human eye, with about 50 percent coming from diffuse sky light, which can reach you even in the shade. According to the Skin Cancer Foundation, to measure your UVB exposure, all you need to do is look up. The amount of UVB you're getting correlates with the amount of sky you can see. If the sky is obstructed by trees or buildings, you're getting less UVB.

Quiz: What Is Your Risk of Getting Sun Damage?

Take this test and find out your danger zone.

1. Tanning is "safe":
    A. When you catch rays only at the tanning salon.
    B. If you tan only when you're on vacation.
    C. Never; there is no such thing as a safe tan.

2. Which of these undesired skin conditions is NOT caused by sun exposure?
    A. Wrinkles
    B. Broken blood vessels
    C. Leprosy

3. Most of the damage we receive from sun exposure is caused:
    A. During our childhood years.
    B. From using baby oil rather than sunscreen.
    C. On that one day on the nude beach.

4. When is the best time to apply sunscreen?
    A. In the morning only.
    B. Thirty minutes before sun exposure and again after swimming or exercise.
    C. About an hour after you've arrived at the beach, when you're just turning pink.

5. If you must be outdoors, try to limit your exposure to:
    A. The hours before 10 A.M. and after 4 P.M.
    B. Only when the kids beg to go to the pool.
    C. Mowing the lawn on weekends.

6. The three main types of skin cancer are:
    A. Basal-cell carcinoma, squamous-cell carcinoma, and malignant melanoma.
    B. Malignant melanoma, keratosis, and warts.
    C. Melanocytic nevus, basal-cell carcinoma, and eczema.

7. What can you wear to minimize sun exposure?
    A. A wide-brimmed hat.
    B. Long-sleeved shirts and long pants.
    C. Tightly woven materials.
    D. All of the above.

8. You don't need to use sunscreen:
    A. On cloudy days.
    B. In the winter.
    C. If you don't mind developing a skin cancer or two.

9. About _____ new cases of skin cancer will be diagnosed in the United States this year:
    A. One hundred thousand.
    B. Five hundred thousand.
    C. One million.

10. The chance of any person developing skin cancer in his or her lifetime is:
    A. Nine out of ten.
    B. One out of six.
    C. Limited only to George Hamilton.

Answers

1. The correct answer is C. There is no such thing as a safe tan. A suntan is the skin's response to an injury; it's what happens as the skin tries to protect itself from further UV damage. A tan is a sign that damage has already been done.

2. The correct answer is C. Okay, this answer was pretty obvious, but did you also know that more than just wrinkles and broken blood vessels are attributable to sun exposure? Try adding dry and leathery skin texture, dull skin tone, age spots, loose skin with poor elasticity, and red blotches. Not a pretty sight!

3. The correct answer is A. Even one bad burn during childhood can set the stage for the development of skin cancer later in life. Keep infants under six months of age out of the sun completely, and apply sunscreen faithfully to all children before any sun exposure.

4. The correct answer is B. Applying sunscreen in the morning is better than not applying it at all—but applying it 30 minutes before leaving your house to go bicycling, swimming, or jogging around the block outdoors will continue your protection. If you waited until you're actually at the beach, by the time you spread out your blanket, put up the umbrella, unpack the cooler, and stop the kids from kicking sand at each other, you'd be red as a lobster.

5. The correct answer is A. The sun's rays are strongest between 10 A.M. and 4 P.M. Whenever possible, try to schedule outdoor activities before or after those hours. When you can't avoid being outside during those hours, make sure you are well protected with sunscreen, hats, and clothing, and try to stay in the shade as much as possible.

6. The correct answer is A. Basal-cell carcinoma is the most commonly occurring skin cancer, followed by squamous-cell, and then malignant melanoma, which is the most deadly.

7. The correct answer is D, all of the above. That was a freebie.

8. The correct answer is C. You can get a serious burn on cloudy days or from the sun's reflection off sand, snow, or even the pavement. What's more, you can get a burn during any season or time of year. That's why it is essential to use a broad-spectrum sunscreen every day.

9. The correct answer is C. According to the American Cancer Society's 1997 projections, more than one million Americans will be diagnosed with some type of skin cancer each year.

10. The correct answer is B. According to the American Academy of Dermatology, at least one in six Americans will develop skin cancer during his or her lifetime.

Score Card

Judge your score by how many questions you answered correctly.

1-3: You probably are burned to a crisp right as we speak. Head out to the drugstore pronto and buy yourself a good sunscreen. Then use it!

4-6: You try to be a savvy consumer, but get confused about what to do, when. Often you lie outside in the sun for hours, thinking that just because you put on an SPF 30, it's okay to soak in the rays. Wrong!

7-9: Aside from getting some incidental exposure while driving or walking, you usually wear sunscreen.

10: A perfect score. You are so health conscious that you must be a doctor.

Did you know that...

Here's another bare truth about sun protection: wearing the right clothes can increase your protection from the sun's damaging rays, which can save you from wrinkles, age spots, and even skin cancer. When you're making clothing picks, choose cotton over silk or wool, a tight weave over a loose weave, dark colors over light colors; and wear a hat with a wide brim.

The Best Way to Use Sunscreen

It might seem simple, but you would be surprised how many people don't know how to put on sunscreen correctly. This is how to do it:

1. Apply your sunscreen at least 20 minutes before sun exposure. This allows the sunscreen to fully absorb into the skin, completely readying the skin to screen out the first ultraviolet rays it encounters.

2. Make sure to use enough sunscreen. One ounce of sunscreen (about one-fourth of most bottles) is adequate to cover all exposed skin. If you don't use enough sunscreen, you won't be able to achieve the SPF rating listed on the product's bottle. In fact, if you use only a small amount of sunscreen, you're likely to cut the SPF rating by half or more, reducing an SPF of 30 to an SPF of 20 or 15, which are still acceptable. However, when a 15 SPF effectively drops to a seven or eight, it may not provide enough protection, especially for people with very fair or sensitive skin.

3. Follow this rule of thumb: even if the label says the product is "waterproof," "sweatproof," or "long-lasting," still reapply it every two hours you stay out in the sun.

4. You must reapply sunscreen immediately after exercising or swimming. Despite manufacturers' claims that certain products are waterproof or sweatproof, no sunscreen is completely sweatproof or waterproof.

5. You also need to apply sunscreen frequently if you participate in outdoor activities, such as tennis, golf, sailing, gardening, horseback riding, etc.

6. Don't make the mistake of using sunscreen as an excuse to lie out in the sun for long periods of time. No matter how much sunscreen you use, you can wind up with more sun damage this way than you would had you lain in the sun for just a short period and gone inside before you started to burn. Sunscreen can be misused by allowing you to stay out for such extended periods of time without early signs of burning that you can end up with ultraviolet damage without realizing it.

7. Throw out your sunscreen after one year, the lifespan of any sunscreen/sunblock product.

Save Your Skin

The key to sun protection could lie in nature and nutrition. Here are some of the latest findings.

Beta Carotene: In the 1950s, researchers found if they added beta carotene to the diets of humans with a genetic disorder that caused them to burn in the sun, they were able to stay out longer without getting burned.

Certain carotenoids (including lycopene and beta carotene) have the ability to increase communication of growth-regulatory signals between cells, which can help prevent damaged cells from becoming cancerous. Still, beta carotene is not yet a replacement for standard sun protection.

Pycnogenol: This French maritime pine-bark extract may be one of the most promising discoveries in the fight against skin cancer. It contains a composite of approximately 40 natural ingredients, including proanthocyanidans, organic acids, and other biologically active components. It works to support the circulatory system by neutralizing the free radicals that attack the body's cells, inhibiting proteolytic enzymes, such as collagenase and elastase, which degrade connective tissue.

Vitamin E: Researchers are examining another potent antioxidant, vitamin E, for its role in sun protection. After UVB irradiation, it appears that the vitamin E concentration in the skin decreases, apparently in response to the increased oxidative stress caused by the free radicals generated by the UV light. Research shows that adding vitamin E to the skin after UV exposure helps the skin to fight sun damage.

Vitamin C: Vitamin C helps neutralize UV-exposure-induced free radicals, which damage collagen, elastin, and other support structures. Free radicals are also thought to produce DNA mutations that can lead to skin cancer. L-ascorbic acid is a water-soluble form of vitamin C thought to help protect skin against UV exposure. A topical formulation was patented by Sheldon Pinnell, M.D., professor of dermatology at Duke University Medical Center in Durham, North Carolina. Pinnell found that L-ascorbic acid applied to the skin before UV exposure could prevent UV-induced immune suppression, which keeps the skin from fighting mutant cells that could turn into skin cancer. Several sunscreen products containing L-ascorbic acid are now on the market.

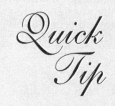

Quick Tip

Avoid wearing perfume while sunbathing. It can cause a photosensitive reaction: dark spots or an itchy rash.

Guerrilla Warfare on Sun-Damaged Skin

Sunscreen: If you do nothing else at all, use a broad-spectrum sunscreen that protects against both UVA and UVB ultraviolet light to help reverse damage and to keep more from occurring.

Glycolic Acid, Amino Fruit Acid, Refinity, Microdermabrasion: Use one of these peels (see Chapter 11) to refresh your skin and remove fine lines and wrinkles. Supplement this with an at-home routine.

Vitamin A: Use vitamin A–derivative products on your skin to reverse sun damage.

Vitamin C: Vitamin C can also help, but it can't be used simultaneously with vitamin A, because C is unstable and when combined with A becomes inactive and no longer works. Sunlight can also inactivate vitamin C, so it's best to use vitamin C (topicals) at night.

Kinerase: This topical cream or lotion, which is derived from plants, helps stimulate fresh collagen and elastin and reduces sun damage. You can get it through your dermatologist.

These next treatments address specific problems that arise after the skin has become damaged by the sun.

Frank Talk on Freckles

Sprinkles of freckles are most often seen on fair-skinned men and women. Although most people think they are a product of genetics, freckles are actually a product of sun damage, most often from the past. Basically, they look like well-defined patches of increased color pigmentation. They differ from moles (see below) in that they do not represent an increased number of pigment, or color, cells, but rather just increased pigmentation, or a darkening in the color, of the skin. You can treat or remove freckles in a number of ways.

How Can I Get Rid of My Freckles?

To get rid of freckles (or at least lighten them up a bit), try using an at-home preparation that has an active lightening ingredient such as hydroquinone, which is available in a 2 percent over-the-counter (Porcelana) or in a 4 percent concentration by prescription (Lustra AF).

Supplement the lightening treatment with products from the vitamin A family, either over-the-counter retinol or prescription agents like Differin, Retin-A, Avita, Renova, and Tazorac. You can also use kojic acid (at home or as part of an office visit), which is derived from a natural substance and is popular in the Far East for its bleaching capabilities, or Azelex cream, which has pigment-correcting properties.

To maximize benefits from any of these products, apply in the morning and leave on the whole day and night, or apply in the evening and leave on until morning.

If this approach doesn't work, try one of the following in-office treatments:

- Glycolic acid peels, amino fruit acid peels, or Refinity facials.
- Beta hydroxy acid peels, such as salicylic acid.
- If none of these treatments work, we step up to microdermabrasion. The next step after that is medium-depth chemical peels or laser resurfacing.
- Whatever treatment you use, continue using sun protection. Otherwise, the freckles more than likely will come right back.

You can zap a single freckle with liquid nitrogen, which is nothing more than nitrogen gas from the atmosphere chilled to freezing. Simply have the dermatologist apply it to the freckle. After a few days, the freckle will scab and fall off. You can also try any of the newer lasers. Both of these procedures can be done fairly quickly and inexpensively, in about five minutes, at a cost of $100 to $500.

Melasma

You can use a lightening agent, such as hydroquinone, in a 4 percent solution, such as Lustra AF, which combines the 4 percent hydroquinone with Parsol 1789 as well as with glycolic acid and topical vitamin C. Another very effective method for fading melasma and freckles is to use topicals from the vitamin A family, such as Avita cream (see Chapter 11).

Moles: Don't Keep Them Underground

Moles on your skin can be annoying. They might not look so great (especially the ones with hair growing out of them) and can make you worry about the state of your health, but most of them are simply annoyances and not life threatening.

Moles are simply well-defined growths in the skin, which can be either flat or raised, pigmented (colored) or nonpigmented (flesh colored), containing hair or hairless. A mole results from the accumulation in a specific area of an increased number of pigment-producing cells (melanocytes), which are normally spread evenly throughout the skin. Melanocytes produce pigment to sustain the skin's normal base color as an overall protection and to increase pigment (tanning) when exposed to the sun. When these cells clump together, they're called moles.

Everyone has at least some moles. The number of moles you develop is determined by a combination of your genetics and your sun exposure, especially during the early years of life. Most people continue to produce new moles through the age of 40 to 45.

Moles can be removed in one of three ways: either by shaving, "burning," or cutting it off. Shaving and "burning" usually require no stitches; cutting a mole out requires stitches to close the incision. Your physician should help you select the most appropriate removal method for the type and location of the mole.

In general, if the mole is suspected to be cancerous, it's probably better to remove it by cutting and stitching, so the pathologist can examine the entire mole.

Currently, no lasers are ideal for removing moles. One problem with lasers that target pigment cells, of which moles are composed, is that they would also remove pigment from the surrounding skin, leaving a lighter area. Another problem is that today's lasers are incapable of completely obliterating all of a mole's color cells. Consequently, it's entirely possible to "zap" a mole with a laser only to later discover, perhaps too late, that the mole had precancerous cells that the procedure either obscured, failed to obliterate, or

Myth:

You don't need a separate sunscreen if your foundation has sunscreen in it.

FACT:

Do you wear foundation on your neck? Your chest? The backs of your hands? Probably not. Plus, many women don't wear foundation every day or all day. Your best bet for effective sun protection to avoid the aging effects of the sun is to apply a sunscreen (or treatment product that contains a sunscreen) to all exposed areas every day.

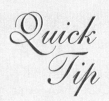

Quick Tip

How long can you safely stay outside? First, ask yourself how quickly you would burn if you weren't wearing any sunscreen (fair-skinned people can burn in as short a period as five minutes). Then, multiply that number by the SPF of whatever product you're using. For example, if you normally start to burn after being in the sun without protection for 10 minutes, a sunscreen with an SPF of 15 allows you to stay out 15 times longer, or a total of 150 minutes, without burning.

stimulated, possibly causing the cancer to spread even further and faster. As advances in technology evolve, newer lasers with the capability to effectively and completely remove unwanted moles will likely emerge.

Fighting Skin Cancer

The best and most important way to fight skin cancer is to make sure you get enough sun protection. As you by now know, there are two predominant wavelengths of ultraviolet light: ultraviolet B (UVB), the short wavelength, and ultraviolet A (UVA), the long wavelength. Most sunscreens protect better against the short wavelength, UVB, but not very well, if at all, against UVA. In fact, the SPF number on the bottle (whether 8, 15, or 30)refers to UVB, not UVA, protection. Problems start when someone applies a high-SPF sunscreen that blocks only UVB and then stays out for prolonged periods of time. This allows more of the weaker, long-wavelength ultraviolet A to penetrate into the skin, damaging the skin cells and increasing the risk of skin cancer.

Confusing News

Some confusing statistics and reports have recently come out about sunscreens. Some statisticians have reported that sunscreens actually increase the risk of skin cancer. This is completely wrong. The only way this can happen is if sunscreen is used improperly.

This misinformation resulted when the statisticians found that both the use of sunscreen and the incidence of skin cancer have increased over the same 10-year period. Their unstudied, unsubstantiated hypothesis: sunscreens must therefore cause skin cancer. This simply isn't true. For one thing, skin cancer takes considerable time to develop and to show up on the skin–up to 50 years.

The only accurate information in the report is the part that says you can get skin cancer if you don't use enough sunscreen or if you stay in the sun too long. The reason is this: although UVA is the weaker of the ultraviolet spectrum, it has a longer wavelength, which dives more deeply into the skin. Here's the kicker: If you used no sunscreen, you normally would get out of the sun when you noticed you were getting sunburned (the effects of UVB rays), which you would notice far sooner than if you were wearing sunscreen. Consequently, you would also get less exposure to UVA rays– which, unlike UVB rays, don't immediately show effects. Because earlier sunscreens targeted UVB, but not UVA, rays, people tended to stay outside in the sun longer before any visible sign of sun exposure appeared. In the process, they also slowly accumulated UVA rays (also very dangerous). It was the misuse of sunscreen and the inaccurate marketing of sunscreen (which gave people a false sense of security, thinking that they could safely spend hours at a time in the sun) that probably caused the increase in skin cancer, not the sunscreen itself.

Check Yourself Out

The other way to attack skin cancer is through routine skin examinations, both at home each month and with your dermatologist, annually. Early detection leads to early removal and cures.

To give yourself a checkup, do the following:

- Examine the entire skin surface. Because skin cancers can arise in areas that get little or no direct sunlight, such as the scalp, between the toes, and the bottoms of the feet, make sure you check out every inch.
- If you find a mole, which is basically a clump of pigment-producing cells, or a growth, ask yourself this question: *Does it look like anything else on my body?* If the answer is yes (meaning, you have other growths that look similar to the one you're wondering about), then it's unlikely what you're looking at represents a skin cancer. Since most people don't develop multiple skin cancers, consider yourself lucky if you find a mate or mates to the spot in question.
- If you're looking at a particular spot or growth and cannot find any other spots or growths on your body that appear similar, then ask yourself: *Is it behaving like other moles or spots on my body?* One of the classic signs of a basal-cell skin cancer, for example, is a sore or "pimple" that doesn't heal. An irregular spot may not be cancerous, but it is definitely cause for suspicion, warranting a trip to the dermatologist.
- Finally, any change (size, color, height, width, texture) in a pre-existing growth or mole requires a trip to the dermatologist. Also, you need to have checked out any mole or growth that becomes itchy, painful, or tingling.

Mole Alert

A mole may be genetic or UV-induced. Although most moles are harmless, some can become cancerous. One way to gauge your risk: if you have more than 10 moles on one of your forearms, you're ten times likelier than the average person to get melanoma.

Jessner's/Efudex

If I find a patient has minor sun damage, I suggest she (or he) follow home treatments and peels to slough off damaged skin, using either vitamin C, vitamin A, or AHAs (see Chapter 11). If I notice the sun damage is more severe and also appears to be potentially precancerous (skin is red, with a slightly rough feeling), I prescribe a series of eight weekly in-office Jessner's/Efudex treatments. The results are nothing short of miraculous.

Efudex was developed as a topical formulation of 5-FU, a standard chemotherapy treatment. It was discovered that chemotherapy treatment with 5-FU caused the precancerous skin cells in patients to disappear along

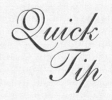

Quick Tip

Got a burn? If you've sprayed yourself with Solarcaine to soothe the pain, it may work wonders, and then again maybe not. Some people are actually allergic to its active ingredient, benzocaine, and often have no clue about their sensitivity, so they respray themselves, causing even more irritation. If Solarcaine worsens your burn, check the ingredients of all topical anesthetics for the suffix "caine" and avoid products that list it.

Quick Tip

- Do not use any form of vitamins C, E, or beta carotene as your sole source of sun protection, because these vitamins do not absorb UV and have no measurable SPF. If you use any of these vitamin products, you must also use a broad-spectrum sunscreen with an SPF of 15 or higher. Until research is conclusive, it's always better to be safe than sorry.

- Retin-A's link to sun sensitivity may be old news, but here's something you probably don't know: After you've used the cream continuously for three months, your body adjusts and becomes more sun-tolerant again. This is good news, but hardly license to stop using sunscreen.

with the cancerous cells. So, the active ingredient 5-FU was formulated into a topical cream, Efudex, to be used at home for two to four weeks. However, the side effects were very unappealing: people using the cream suffered from crusty, oozing, inflamed skin as the formula worked its way through the skin's layers. Because of the unsightly side effects, many people decided not to use it. That problem led the Columbia University Dermatology Department to come up with alternative ways to use Efudex. Through research a procedure was developed that worked: Jessner's solution, a mild exfoliant, was used in combination with a liquid form of Efudex to target precancerous cells. The Efudex with Jessner's solution formulation works because the exfoliant loosens the protein bonds between the cells of the top skin layer, so that when the liquid Efudex is applied minutes later, it easily penetrates into the damaged tissue, breaking apart microscopic layers of cells. To illustrate this concept, picture a brick or concrete wall. Then, imagine what happens when someone pours a pitcher of water across the top. It doesn't get through. However, if there are hairline cracks in the surface of the block, the water is able to trickle through. That's what the Jessner's does: it creates microscopic cracks that enable the Efudex to work, killing precancerous skin cells, while leaving healthy ones.

My patients love the results. After just eight sessions (once weekly), for about $150 per treatment, the precancerous cells are gone, the pigmentation color is even, and the skin looks healthy and glowing.

Self-Tanning Talk

I've been suggesting all along that the best tan isn't a natural tan. A tan from a bottle works just fine. Self-tanners contain DHA (dihydroxyacetone), derived from sugar, which works by staining the skin. Here are a few application tips:

- Before applying tanner, exfoliate in the shower, using a washcloth, and then smooth on some moisturizer.
- Try to match the tanner to your skin tone. If you're fair-skinned, go for a light label; if you're olive-skinned, try a medium; and if you're in the bronze/brown zone, go for the dark. Try to stay away from extra-dark formulas, which can leave most skins looking orangey.
- Choose products that instantly deposit color on the skin, so you can catch any areas you missed instantly.
- Wait a while after showering to self-tan. The heat in the shower causes your pores to dilate, which can make your tanner streak. Instead, take a break and wait about 20 minutes.

Products to try:

For oily skin, choose light, nongreasy, noncomedogenic formulas like Clarins Gel Auto-Bronzant Self Tanning Gel or Coppertone Oil-Free Sunless Tanner.

For dry skin, get tanners with moisturizing ingredients, like those found in Bath & Body Works Moisturizing Sunless Tanner. For sensitive, dry skin, try mild, hypoallergenic products such as Physicians Formula Sun Shield, Sears Circle of Beauty Skinplicity, and Neutrogena Sunless Tanning Spray.

Common Questions

Q: Is it true that in terms of sun protection, anything over SPF 15 doesn't count?

A: This is not necessarily true, especially for people who have lighter or more sensitive skin or for people who are out in the sun for an extended period of time. For those people, products that have a higher SPF (sun protection factor) can make a difference. For example, an SPF of 15 blocks approximately 93 percent of the ultraviolet rays, while an SPF of 30 may block 97 percent. This can make the difference between a sunburn for a person with light or sensitive skin.

Q: I like to go to tanning salons to get a little color before the summer begins. I've heard that some salons have beds that emit only UVA radiation, which doesn't burn you as fast. Are they safer?

A: Absolutely not. Some men and women put sunscreen on and then go off to tanning parlors. This makes no sense to me at all. It's a complete contradiction of terms. It reminds me of a person who smokes while jogging on a track. There is no safe tan, contrary to what tanning salons might want you to believe. All tanning beds use UVA rays, which actually cause more damage than other types of rays, because they have a longer wavelength and penetrate deep into the dermis. UVA rays break down the skin's elastic structures and will eventually make you more wrinkly and leathery than tanning outdoors would.

I have seen an increase in melanoma in young women in their twenties and thirties, and I feel this is partly due to increased use of tanning beds. I always tell my patients that if they have to tan, I would rather they do it outside.

Did you know that...

- Most cotton T-shirts block only 50 percent of the sun's rays. In fact, according to the Skin Cancer Foundation, light cotton T-shirts and polo shirts typically have an SPF of only 6 or 7, which is far below the recommended SPF of 15. Rule of thumb: What you can see through, UV light can get through. If your shirt gets wet, it blocks less—only 30 to 40 percent—of UV rays.
- Hats don't take the place of a sunblock, since most ultraviolet rays bounce off of the ground, pavement, or snow.
- Color-treated hair is likely to get bleached (not to mention fried) from the sun. To protect: Comb conditioner with SPF through wet hair; you can substitute sunscreen in a pinch.
- Lips contain little melanin, which makes it impossible for them to tan. However, the lack of melanin also makes it easy for them to burn. Slick lips with an SPF-containing lip balm throughout the day to keep them smooth.

The bottom line: damaged skin is damaged skin, and a tan is a sign your cells have been injured. Places may advertise that their machines reach Food and Drug Administration standards. But the FDA officially discourages the use of sunlamps. In fact, when it says FDA approved, it simply means the FDA has approved the tanning beds (the equipment), not the procedure per se. It means, in effect, that the equipment operates as it should, and the top won't fall down and break your head. At tanning parlors, you get high-energy UVA, so you are better off outside in the regular sun, because the UVB doesn't penetrate the skin so deeply.

Q: Is it safe to use last year's sunscreen?

A: As long as it's no more than a year old (the shelf-life of most sunscreens). However, if you notice a change in color, a bad smell, or some clumping, or if you feel a burning sensation after applying it, you should dump it. These are signs that the active ingredients are no longer capable of absorbing UV light.

Q: My self-tanner came out all splotchy looking. How can I correct it?

A: Whatever you do, don't reapply the self-tanner to fill in the light spots; it'll just make more of an unsightly mess. Instead, you need to remove the self-tanner you've already put on by exfoliating with a body scrub every day for the next few days. Try to be gentle (you don't want to rub your skin raw). After a few days, reapply the tanner, but first mix it with a little moisturizer, so your skin won't absorb quite so much of it. This will also help even out the overall color.

Q: Will swimming in a chlorinated pool hurt my skin?

A: Not necessarily. Since chlorine contains antibacterial ingredients, it can actually be beneficial to people with oily skin or acne. But chlorine can be drying to normal or sensitive skin. If your skin feels tight after swimming, rinse off in a warm shower, then slather a rich moisturizing lotion all over your body.

Q: I'm only 22 years old, but I've been a sun worshipper (oils, reflecting mirrors) since I was a young teen. I always love the way I look with a tan, and I don't have any wrinkles yet. How can I tell whether I have sun damage?

A: You can look at your skin under something called a Wood's lamp, which projects a long wavelength of ultraviolet light deeper into skin than visible light. If you have sun damage (and you probably do), it'll show up as heavy freckling all over. Clumps that show up under the lamp mean that you are in the early stages of sun damage, wherein the skin's pigment-producing cells, called melanocytes, lose their ability to distribute pigment evenly. As the damage proliferates, your face will show it in the form of a duller complexion, freckles, blotches, visible blood vessels, and wrinkles. As the years progress—and if you don't stop the damage and get your "tan" from a self-tanning bottle, instead—you'll look wrinkly, leathery, and possibly get skin cancer.

Q: What can I do if I get sunburned?

A: Try these treatments:

- Apply moisturizer.
- If you know you've had too much sun, take Tylenol or Advil quickly, because it can diminish the sunburn reaction on the skin.
- Avoid taking cold baths or showers.
- Drink plenty of water to offset dehydration.
- If it's a bad burn, get to your dermatologist.

Q: I take medication. Should I worry about going out into the sun?

A: You should check your medication type, warnings, and side effects. Some over-the-counter prescriptions are photosensitizers, meaning they change chemically when exposed to UV rays and can cause sunburns, rashes, swelling, and allergic reactions. These include the following:

- Ibuprofen makes you especially susceptible to sunburn. For safer relief of cramps or pain, take aspirin or acetaminophen.
- Doxycycline, the antibiotic most often prescribed for Lyme disease, is also a well-known sun sensitizer.
- To be extra safe, check with your doctor or pharmacist when taking medication and going out in the sun.

Myth: Self-tanners turn on the body's own melanin, or pigment production.

FACT: Self-tanners have no effect on melanin production. The active ingredient in over-the-counter self-tanners is DHA (dihydroxy acetone), a noncarcingenic (not cancer-causing) derivative of sugar cane. These products do not cause a true "tan." When the dihydroxy acetone reacts on the skin, it produces a brownish color, essentially a temporary stain, that gives the appearance of a tan. But this "tan" doesn't turn on, or increase, the body's own melanin, or pigment, production—which is what happens with a sun-induced tan—nor does it provide the sun protection of a true tan. This leads to a potential problem: Some people who apply self-tanners may mistakenly think they have a base tan that will protect them; then when they go out in the sun, they can get a nasty sunburn. That is why it is important to use a self-tanner with an SPF 15 or higher or to also apply sunscreen. Newer self-tanner products are very good and don't stain your skin orange, which the first generation of products tended to do.

chapter thirteen

Body Talk

We are born naked, wet, and hungry.
Then things get worse.
—BUMPER STICKER

YOUR SKIN TAKES UP 1.73 SQUARE METERS TO STRETCH OVER YOUR FLESH AND BONES, so you want to baby it from head to toe. Here is an A to Z primer on tending all of your parts. Later in this chapter I'll provide you with information on other important body care topics, such as hair removal techniques, answers to your most common skin care questions, and research that shows the positive impact of fitness on your skin—and on your life.

Baby Your Body

Here are some simple recommendations for exfoliating, moisturizing, treating, and enhancing your different body areas.

Arms

Some women tend to get chicken skin, called keratosis pilaris, on their upper arms. These little bumps resemble the ones you get on your butt. Try using a lotion containing AHAs or BHAs to slough them off. However, be careful with your scrubbing tool—using a loofah or a grainy scrub may feel good temporarily, but may actually worsen the condition.

Back

Backs and shoulders often break out. To prevent nasty eruptions:

*   Wash daily, and gently use a soft-bristled scrub brush.

161

- Fight blackheads with a mild salicylic acid cleanser or dab on a 2.5 to 10 percent benzoyl peroxide treatment (go to 10 percent only if skin is oily and not irritated by the concentration).
- Make sure to shower promptly after exercising to remove sweat and oils.

Breasts

Your décolleté and breasts have very few sebaceous glands (unlike your upper chest), so they tend to get dry. To keep them moist and to avoid ugly patches of dry skin:

- Moisturize after bathing or showering.
- Soothe chafed nipples (from jogging, breastfeeding, working out) with a thin film of petroleum jelly or Aquaphor moisturizer. Cover with an old bra. Check first with your pediatrician or OB/GYN if you are breastfeeding.

Elbows

Almost everyone has complaints about these rough spots. That's because the skin's top layer of dead cells is thicker on elbows than anywhere else on the body. To keep them smooth:

- Apply a thick moisturizer often.
- Try a 12 percent AHA product (Am-Lactin over the counter).
- Wash with an alpha hydroxy cleanser and exfoliate several times a week.

Feet

It's easy to overlook feet, but you shouldn't. Foot problems can be quite painful, but they are easily prevented. To keep feet in fighting shape:

- Cleanse them daily.
- Remove dead skin with a pumice stone (or use an exfoliant).
- Clip toenails short and straight to prevent ingrown toenails.
- Wear shoes that fit well, are comfortable, and don't squeeze your feet or toes.
- If you get nail fungus, treat it with either topical or oral medications.
- Treat athlete's foot with a medicated powder.
- Check for warts, and if you have one, see a dermatologist—otherwise, it may spread and/or grow.
- Wear sunblock all over your feet (heels included). A sunburn on the tops or the soles of the feet hurts!

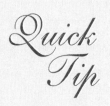

Quick Tip

When it comes to bathing, you should choose between two options: Take either a short warm or a long warm bath. The reason? Excessive bathing can dry out your skin, but a quick bath won't. If you take a long bath, you can superhydrate your skin. The problem, however, occurs with taking a bath of medium duration, say, 15 to 20 minutes. Why? Because with a medium-length bath, the rate of evaporation may exceed the rate of hydration, and you'll wind up drying out your skin.

Hands

An old saying says, "You can tell a woman's true age by her hands." In many ways, that is still true. Many women (and men) don't take care of their hands, at least not as well as they take care of their faces, and the aging skin really shows it.

The skin on the hands is subject to the same damaging effects of the sun and environment as is the face, especially since you rarely cover them (except in the coldest weather). Hands also rarely reap the soothing benefits of moisturizers and sunscreens that you give the rest of your body. Even more wearing is that your hands endure the harsh treatment of repeated hand washings (which can dry them out) and that they touch paper and other harsh materials all day long (which is doubly drying to hands). Start treating your hands well by treating them the same way you would treat your face:

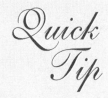

Quick Tip

For a hands-on guide to treating your hands right, why not ask a hand model? Ellen Sirot of Parts Models offers these additional tips to keeping your hands soft and supple:

- Apply vitamin E oil to cuticles every night.

- Use a soft-bristled nail brush to clean under nails when you wash your hands.

- Push back cuticles with a washcloth in the shower.

- Use rich moisturizers, vitamin A products, glycolic acid products, vitamin C products, and peeling treatments.
- Always wear sunscreen to prevent "age" and "liver" spots, which are all directly caused by sun exposure. Hands get extra sun exposure, believe it or not, from their position on the wheel when you're driving your car; the backs of your hands get all the sun's damaging rays right through the windshield. Use a higher-SPF sunscreen (as you should on the rest of your body) when you will be exposed to direct sun for extended periods of time.
- When you wash your hands, use the mildest antibacterial cleanser you can find.
- Wear gloves when washing dishes (hot water is very drying to all skin).
- Put your face cream products on your hands at night to get great results. (Because you don't wash your hands while you sleep, the products will have the greatest amount of time to penetrate.)

Knees

- Wash your knees with alpha hydroxy acid–containing products.
- Apply a thick moisturizer, such as Curél Concentrated Moisturizing Cream.
- Use a 12 percent AHA prescription product, such as Lac-Hydrin.
- Try using an exfoliating mask on built-up dead skin on knees.

Hair, Hair, Go Away

So many methods of hair removal are available today that it's easy to get a smooth face and body. Here are some of the most common methods:

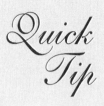

Quick Tip

Beware of taking a long soak in a tub filled with bubble bath. Most bubble bath products contain a solvent detergent, which is abrasive on skin (not to mention on your nether parts). It's kind of like putting yourself in a washing machine. If you insist on doing it, use a rich moisturizer all over as soon as you dry yourself off.

Shaving—A Quick and Easy Way to Hair-Free Skin

- Moisten hairs before shaving. Otherwise, you'll get razor burn.
- Lather on a shave cream or gel, and let it sit for a few minutes.
- Never exfoliate or apply AHA lotions right after shaving—it will sting!
- Change blades often. They become dull after five to seven shaves.
- Shave against the direction of hair growth. That's how you'll get the closest shave. If your skin is very sensitive, shave with the direction of the hair growth.
- Avoid shaving right before swimming. Chlorine and salt water can sting freshly shaved skin, causing irritation.

Waxing

Waxing is most often done at a salon. It can also be done with a do-it-at-home kit.

Don't wax the week before or during your period, when you retain water and skin is more sensitive.

Don't wax if you are taking Accutane or using topical vitamin A products—you can rip off a layer of skin.

Regrowth occurs in three to six weeks. Loofahs or body scrubs between waxings help prevent ingrowns. Pluck off some stubble from shorter hairs.

Depilatories

These hair-removal preparations are quick, painless, and come in different formulations, depending on where they are used: face or body. They remove hair below the skin's surface, and it lasts for about two weeks.

If you have sensitive skin, acne, sunburn, or hives, exercise caution when using depilatories; the chemicals can cause a mild reaction or some burning.

Electrolysis and Lasers

For a complete description of laser hair removal, see Chapter 14.

Stressed Out? Get a Massage

Who doesn't love a massage when they are tense? However, using oils for your massage can block your pores and contribute to breakouts. Many of my patients complain when the beneficial, pleasurable aspects of a massage are minimized by pimples and cysts that occur several days after the massage. To solve this dilemma, I instruct patients to have massages with oil-free moisturizers, such as Neutrogena, Purpose, or Complex-15, instead of with oils. Most masseurs are happy to comply, and the patient's pores remain unblocked and blemish-free.

A COMPARISON OF HAIR REMOVAL METHODS

METHOD	ADVANTAGE	DISADVANTAGE
Laser	Permanent Changes the quality and texture of the hair Regrows thinner in diameter and lighter in color	Some skin irritation Costly initially
Electrolysis	Long-term results	Painful, invasive procedure that requires the insertion of a needle into individual hair follicles Works best on upper lip, eyebrows, and other problem areas Only treats one hair follicle at a time Expensive Requires numerous visits Can cause scarring May cause skin irritation (especially if needle is too hot)
Waxing	Quick and easy Can be done at home	Painful Short-term results (4–6 weeks) Invasive, rips hair from roots Can get ingrown hairs Can cause skin irritation Can cause inflammation of the hair follicle
Sugaring	Quick and easy Can be done at home	Best if done at a salon (a mix of sugar and lemon is applied and flicked off, removing hair at the roots) May be painful
Depilatory	Quick and easy Can be done at home	May be painful Can burn skin Lasts 2–4 weeks Can cause irritation and dryness Unpleasant smell
Shaving	Quick and easy Can be done anywhere Less trauma to the skin than other methods Doesn't make hair coarser or thicker	Must repeat often Can get ingrown hairs Can irritate skin Only removes hair from the surface of the skin, doesn't treat the follicle directly.

Common Questions

Q: I tend to bite my cuticles. Is there a cure? And what can I do to make my nails look good?

A: You probably follow a pattern: You get stressed, bite your cuticles, and then get stressed again when you see how bad your nails look (dry, ragged, peeling). That just makes you start biting again. Stop the insanity! Start by washing your hands with an antibacterial soap and soaking them in warm water. Then remove any hangnails with a cuticle nipper. Follow with a cuticle oil or a rich hand cream to keep cuticles smooth and moisturized. Get into the habit of applying the cream daily, and you'll begin to take pride in your nails, instead of taking a bite out of them.

Q: Why do I get goose bumps?

A: Goose bumps appear on the skin as tiny muscles contract. It's a way for the body to expose a smaller surface area to the cold and to make hair stand on end for better insulation.

Q: I'm worried about getting acne from sweating when I work out. What should I do?

A: When you work out, skip the makeup. The combination of sweat and makeup can clog your pores and block the evaporation of sweat, leading to breakouts. Wear a sweatband to keep hair off your face. Also wear moisture-wicking fabrics on underpants and feet (such as CoolMax and Dri-FIT) to avoid creating a bacteria-friendly environment. Also, always shower immediately after working out.

Q: Is it okay to use products that claim they are "all natural"?

A: Many products claim they have "all natural ingredients" and are, therefore, good for you. That isn't always the case. Just remember, poison ivy, snake venom, salmonella, porcupines, and lightning are "all natural"–and I certainly wouldn't want to come into contact with any of them!

Q: I'm bored with soap and want to try out one of the new shower gels. Is it worth it?

A: Many of the shower gels are nice smelling, but a lot of them are heavily fragranced, which is the leading cause of skin allergies. Many of them come with material buff puff scrubbers, which can get bacteria overgrowth. Also, consider the cost. How many showerings do you get out of a bottle of these cleansers versus a much cheaper bar of fragrance-free soap?

Q: I work out often, and I feel like my skin is getting dehydrated. I apply moisturizer, but I still have the problem.

A: Are you taking two showers a day now (one at home and one at the gym, where the liquid cleansers are as strong as industrial detergents)? That may be the cause. To prevent the problem, bring your own moisturizing soap to the gym, and don't lather your whole body, only where you really need cleansing. Make sure the water temperature is not too hot (which can strip your skin of its natural oils). Of course, once you get out of the shower, apply moisturizer directly onto damp skin (to seal in the water).

Q: I shower and use deodorant every day, but in the summer I tend to smell. What should I do?

A: When the temperature and the humidity level soar, it's easy to smell bad. To fix:

- Shower daily with antibacterial soap.
- After showering, wait at least 15 minutes and then apply a deodorant/antiperspirant to dry underarms. Put it on at bedtime, too, for more drying power.
- Shave your armpits, which are breeding grounds for bacteria, as soon as you see stubble.
- Avoid wearing tight tops; wear loose cotton clothing.
- Stick with natural over artificial fibers. (Natural fibers breathe; artificial fibers lock in wetness.)
- If you've tried everything, check with your doctor. He may prescribe either an antibiotic cleanser or an antiperspirant deodorant, like Drysol. You may also have a hormonal condition.

Did you know that…

- The skin is the largest organ system of the body. It consists of three layers: The epidermis (the outer layer), the dermis (connective tissue), and the subcutis (fat layer).

- It covers and protects the internal organs, acts as a barrier to external contaminants and injury, helps prevent dehydration, is a sensory organ, and helps regulate body temperature.

- You are born with approximately 100,000 hair follicles on your scalp. Baldness and hair loss happen when the hair follicles "poop" out.

- It takes three to six months to grow out a fingernail and 12 to 18 months to grow out a toenail.

Q: I tend to have dry, flaky patches on my skin. Someone suggested I get a humidifier. Will that help me?

A: A humidifier can help, because it adds more moisture to the air. You can also try placing a pan full of water (warm) on the radiator for the same effect. If you buy a humidifier, make sure to clean it often, since you don't want bacteria to be released into the air.

Q: Is it okay to use some of the new fancy face products on my back, hands, and other parts of my body?

A: There are several new products that have special qualities, including:

- Beaded Scrubs: Tiny collapsible beads in cleansers that help to exfoliate skin. Try Neutrogena's New Pore-Refining Cream or Bioré Mild Daily Cleansing Scrub.
- Pore Strips: Adhesive strips that latch on to blackheads, dirt, and dead skin cells and lift them off for a temporary fix for clogged pores. Try Neutrogena Deep Clean Pore Strips, Bioré Warming Deep Pore Cleanser, or Almay's StayClean Medicated Pore Strips (which contain salicylic acid).
- Oil Blotters and Towelettes: These remove makeup and dirt, using cleansers, alcohol, and water. You can pack them in a bag for travel, and they don't spread bacteria. Because the ingredients are mild, they work for all skin types.

chapter fourteen

A Look at Lasers

*In the depths of winter I finally learned there
was in me an invincible summer.*
—Albert Camus

THERE IS NO BETTER TOOL TO USE TO ZAP CERTAIN ANNOYING PARTS OF YOUR SKIN,
while leaving others alone, than lasers. Although you may think "Star Wars" when
you look at a laser, they have actually been used by dermatologists for nearly forty
years. Lasers aren't magic, but in the hands of a skilled doctor, they can be the cure
to what ails you. Before you sign up for a laser treatment, make sure to ask the
doctor a few hard questions:

Question Corner
Ask the doctor:

> "How many laser treatments have you performed?"
> "Can I see before and after photos of patients?"
> "Can I speak to some of your patients?" (patients who have had the same treat-
> ment you are considering)

You may also want to ask the doctor what has been the worst complication
he/she has ever faced during a treatment and how it was resolved.

In dermatology, lasers are used for different purposes: skin resurfacing (to
improve scars, lines and wrinkles, and sun damage), treating broken blood vessels,
warts, removing tattoos, and hair removal. Here's a guide to the wonderful world
of lasers and what the right one can do for you.

Resurfacing Lasers
What They Are Good For: Skin resurfacing with a laser effectively removes superficial sun damage in the form of age spots and other pigmentation, smooths out

169

lines and wrinkles, and improves scars, such as from acne or chicken pox. Two different kinds of lasers are the carbon dioxide, or CO_2 laser, and the Erbium:YAG laser.

Benefits: Both have the same skin-smoothing and rejuvenating effect.

- The CO_2 laser works particularly well for deep wrinkles and scars. The Erbium is a cooler laser than the CO_2, meaning that it beams less heat into the skin. Therefore, the level of depth is more controllable, hence the "damage" to the skin can be more limited and can be performed under local anesthesia, whereas the CO_2 laser frequently requires general anesthesia or intravenous sedation.
- Recovery time is fast; three to seven days for the Erbium and 7 to 14 days for the CO_2. As the skin heals, it goes from a dark to a light pink color that fades rapidly over several weeks after Erbium resurfacing; after CO_2, pinkness can take 3 to 6 months to fade.
- As the skin heals, there is a tightening effect and the production of fresh collagen is stimulated, so the skin becomes healthier and better-looking than it was before.
- Resurfacing lasers surpass many facial treatments used in the past. The concept is simple: A laser is used to remove the damaged outer layers of skin to allow the skin underneath to grow new, healthier layers of skin. No other procedure can match the dramatic results of laser resurfacing with as little downtime.
- Resurfacing can also be performed on other areas of the body, such as the chest or the backs of hands.

Weaknesses: Laser resurfacing is laser resurfacing. No matter which you choose, you must deal with a period where your skin is raw and oozing. However, as I've just mentioned, you can't beat the results.

Cost: $2,000 for either the area around the mouth or the area around the eyes.
$5,000 for the full face.

My personal favorite and the laser I use for resurfacing in my practice is the Erbium:YAG laser because of its efficiency and quicker healing time. The Erbium allows the doctor to focus on the affected skin layers, leaving the underlying layers virtually untouched. It can be used without sedation, just topical anesthetic. Because the Erbium creates less tissue damage and has less heat than the CO_2, it's better for treating localized areas on the face, such as just around the mouth or just around the eyes, which heal without the color blending problems that can occur with the CO_2. Best of all, even a patient who undergoes resurfacing on her entire face is back in the swing of things, with a little cover-up makeup, in about a week or so.

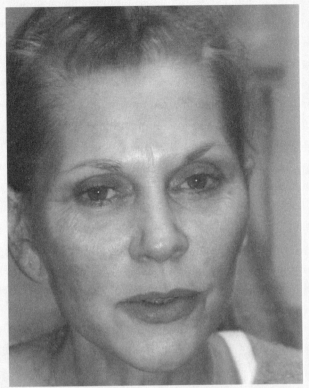

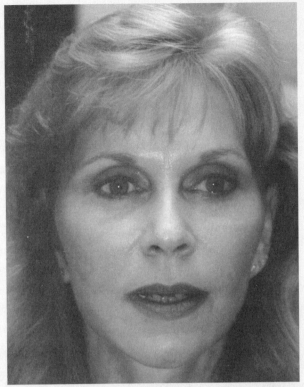

BEFORE: 52-YEAR-OLD WOMAN BEFORE FULL FACE LASER RESURFACING

AFTER: PATIENT THREE MONTHS AFTER LASER RESURFACING WITH THE ERBIUM: YAG LASER. NOTE SKIN TIGHTENING EFFECT OF LASER RESURFACING.

Name: KR
Age: 52

PROBLEM:	Sun-damaged skin and fine lines and wrinkles that wouldn't disappear, despite good skin care.
SHE WANTED:	Dramatic results. A colleague of mine says, "If you want dramatic results, you have to do something dramatic," and this patient was willing to go for it.
HER CONCERNS:	What the recuperation period would be like.
DOCTOR'S ADVICE:	Laser resurfacing would give her the results she was looking for: smoother, brighter skin with less sun damage. In a week or so, she could use camouflaging makeup and return to work.
WHAT SHE HAD DONE:	Erbium:YAG laser resurfacing of her entire face.
HER REACTION:	She is very happy with her appearance and the compliments she (still) receives from friends and even strangers, who can't believe she is 52.

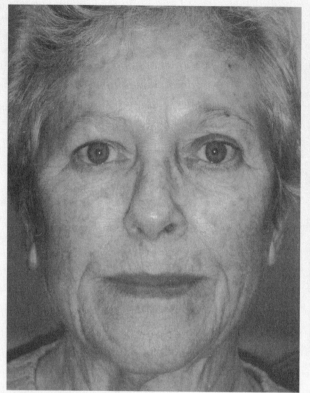
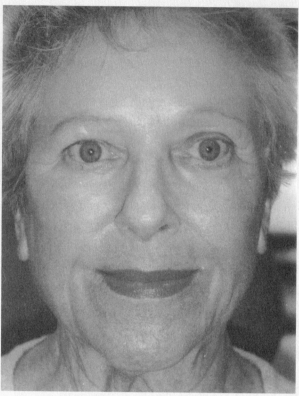

BEFORE: 69-YEAR-OLD WOMAN BEFORE FULL FACE ERBIUM LASER RESURFACING.

AFTER: PATIENT TWO WEEKS AFTER PROCEDURE WITH NO MAKEUP EXCEPT LIPSTICK. NOTE DRAMATIC SKIN TIGHTENING AFTER LASER RESURFACING.

Name: LB
Age: 69

PROBLEM:	Moderate to severe wrinkles and sun damage.
WHAT SHE WANTED:	An improvement in all of the above.
HER CONCERNS:	Was a face-lift appropriate, or was there another procedure she could have done?
DOCTOR'S ADVICE:	A face-lift, although it would smooth out wrinkles, would do nothing for the quality of the skin itself and therefore would have no impact on the sun damage.
WHAT SHE HAD DONE:	A full-face Erbium:YAG laser resurfacing.
HER REACTION:	She was so happy with the results that she brought in her sister from Florida to get the same procedure.

A Word of Caution

If you are considering laser resurfacing, your most important consideration is to have the procedure done by a very seasoned, experienced practitioner who has performed many, many of these treatments with whichever laser he/she is recommending. Of all the lasers in dermatology, the resurfacing lasers probably present the greatest potential for scarring and infection if something goes wrong.

Lasers to Treat Broken Blood Vessels

This class of laser treats broken blood vessels, either on the face or any other part of the body, including spider veins on the legs. These lasers also treat the little red dots known as angiomas and raised red spots or birthmarks known as hemangiomas. They all work by passing through the skin's surface and the laser beam is selectively absorbed by the red blood cells below, causing them to rupture (which is harmless) and then be reabsorbed by the body. Because the laser goes right through the skin's surface, it causes no break or disruption of the outer surface at all. All cause some degree of redness afterward. Because there are more lasers in this category and each has it's distinctive features, I've listed them separately below.

Pulsed Dye Laser

The Pulsed Dye Laser is, in my opinion, the best of this category. It works well for eliminating broken blood vessels, port-wine stains, small spider veins, stretch marks, and elevated scars (above the skin's surface) such as hypertrophic scars. It is also effective in treating warts by cutting off blood supply to the wart.

Benefits:

* It is the most efficient of all these lasers for long-term elimination of broken blood vessels.
* There is no scabbing, crusting, or oozing and therefore no chance of infection.
* It can reduce diffuse pink or redness across the central face that is often associated with rosacea, a condition characterized by diffuse redness on both cheeks and across the nose.
* It can reduce the appearance of scars and stretch marks (although it is most effective when the area is still pink, as opposed to older and faded to white).

Weaknesses:

* Pulsed dye laser treatments cause a purple bruising at the site of the treated area that can last anywhere from several days to one or two weeks and can be difficult to camouflage with makeup. Because of this bruising, make sure to discuss your schedule with your doctor and your

potential for downtime. It is not physically uncomfortable but some people are self-conscious about being seen in public with this kind of result.

Cost: $1,500 for a full face.

$500 per treatment for leg veins (requires one to three treatments).

$250 and up for warts.

$250 and up for a small area of broken blood vessels, scar, or stretch marks.

Krypton Laser

The krypton laser is good for treating broken blood vessels and angiomas anywhere on the body.

Benefits:

- This laser has been around for many years and is very safe.
- It does not cause bruising but a little inflammation that heals quickly, usually in a few days.

Weaknesses:

- It is less effective at treating diffuse areas and impractical for treating large areas of pink or red.
- Not as effective at long-term eradication of broken blood vessels.

Cost: $500 per treatment.

VersaPulse Laser

The VersaPulse laser does a good job on broken blood vessels, spider veins, and removing tattoos.

Benefits:

- This is a relatively newer laser that avoids the bruising you get with the pulsed dye laser.

Weaknesses:

- Like the krypton laser, not effective on diffuse areas of pink or red.
- Also not as effective for long-term eradication of broken blood vessels.

Cost: $200 to $1,000 for broken blood vessels on face.

$500 for spider veins.

$350 per each 15 minute session for tattoos.

Argon Laser

Benefit:

- This is an older technology that is effective at treating well-defined, individual broken blood vessels.

Weakness:

* Some scarring has been associated with the argon laser. Therefore only an experienced clinician should perform this treatment.

Cost: $500 per treatment.

Intense Pulsed Light

Not really lasers but intense pulsed light, these are used in many leg vein centers and are also used for hair removal. Two models by the same company are called EpiLight and PhotoDerm.

Cost: $500 per treatment.

Quick Note on Spider Veins

For the treatment of leg veins, most doctors still consider injections, or sclerotherapy, to be the gold standard or treatment of choice for most leg veins, for several reasons. Only the tiniest spider veins are effectively treated with lasers; larger vessels do not respond particularly well to current light sources. Contrary to popular belief, sclerotherapy is often less uncomfortable than lasers. Injections cause minimal bruising or discoloration, whereas laser therapy commonly causes more bruising and discoloration that, although also temporary, can last longer.

Hair Removal Lasers

In the age-old quest to remove unwanted body hair, lasers are the newest entry into the arsenal. In the short time since they have been used for this purpose, this category has seen many laser manufacturers try for the coveted ability to claim permanent results. In an effort to cause the hair to not regrow, most of the lasers work on the same principle of targeting dark pigment, or melanin. Because of this, many of these lasers are mentioned again in the pigment removing category, but keep in mind that although they have the same name, they are different lasers at different settings to achieve different results.

Diode Laser

This is the only laser to receive FDA clearance in its claim of permanent results for hair removal. This laser requires a series of three to six treatments, at approximately four- to eight-week intervals, to achieve significant, permanent hair reduction. It is the only laser designed specifically and solely for the purpose of hair removal. This laser cannot be used if you are tan, however, because it will target that pigmentation. For that reason, it is less effective than some others for both fair-haired and dark-skinned patients. The LightSheer laser is a diode system, and it offers a cool tip to reduce discomfort.

Cost: $250 to $700 per treatment, per body area.

Did you know that...

The ancient Egyptians considered body hair unhygienic and used many traditional methods of hair removal, including razors, tweezers, and combs.

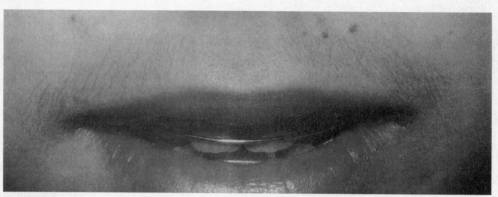

BEFORE: 15-YEAR-OLD GIRL BEFORE LASER HAIR REMOVAL ON UPPER LIP.

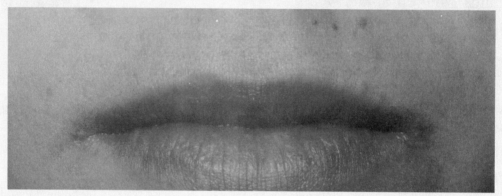

AFTER: PATIENT SIX MONTHS AFTER LASER TREATMENT. NOTE VIRTUAL ABSENCE OF HAIR REGROWTH.

Name: CM

Age: 15

PROBLEM:	Troublesome hair on her upper lip.
WHAT SHE WANTED:	To get rid of it!
HER CONCERNS:	Would it work and would it hurt?
DOCTOR'S ADVICE:	A topical numbing cream takes care of the discomfort, and the new LightSheer Diode laser is showing permanent results after at least three treatments.
WHAT SHE HAD DONE:	LightSheer Diode laser treatment on her upper lip.
HER REACTION:	She's much less aware about the hair now and is glad she no longer faces years of waxing or other tedious methods of hair removal.

Neodymium (Nd) YAG Laser (long pulse)

This is the laser used in the Thermolase SoftLight system. It works in conjunction with a topically applied carbon lotion to target hair follicles. Its strength is that it can treat all hair and skin types; its weakness is that usually more treatments are needed and the hair reduction is short-lived.

Cost: $150 to $500 per treatment, per body part.

Alexandrite (long pulse)

Like the Nd YAG laser, the Alexandrite laser can be used to successfully remove unwanted hair in darker-skinned patients without a loss of pigmentation. This is the laser used in the GentleLase and EpiTouch (Alexandrite) systems.

Cost: $250 to $700 per treatment, per body part.

Q-Switched Ruby Laser

This laser is used less these days because of its limitations. It is more likely to cause loss of pigmentation than some other lasers, is effective only for patients with pale skin and dark hair, and has a slightly higher incidence of blistering.

Cost: $250 to $700 per treatment, per body part.

Intense Pulsed Light

As mentioned before, these are not really lasers but can be used for hair removal by targeting dark pigment in the hair follicle.

Cost: $250 to $700 per treatment, per body part.

Electrolysis

This is also not a laser but is a hair removal system and worth mentioning here. Electrolysis sends an electric pulse down each individual hair shaft (one hair at a time) to shock the hair follicle and inhibit regrowth. It is time consuming and impractical for large areas, but less expensive and therefore cost effective for areas where the hair density is sparse. Laser hair removal is more expensive than electrolysis, but is 60 times faster and less painful than electrolysis; also, fewer sessions are needed with the laser with better results.

Cost: Approximately $30 for 30 minutes, enough time to treat an upper lip.

Lasers for Tattoo and Pigment Removal

As mentioned before, some of the same types of lasers that work for hair removal are also used to remove tattoos and pigmented lesions, such as solar lentigines or café-au-lait spots. Again, they work on different wavelengths and are different lasers. Here are the lasers and which color pigments they are used to treat:

Nd YAG	Blue, black, green, red, yellow, orange, brown, dark brown
Alexandrite	Black, blue, and especially effective for green
Ruby	Purple, violet, other dark colors but particularly black. Will not remove red
Pulsed dye	Red, orange, and yellow

What do I think is the best laser for each purpose?

Laser resurfacing for wrinkles and/or sun damage–Erbium:YAG laser
Laser resurfacing for scars–Erbium:YAG and/or pulsed dye laser
Broken blood vessels–pulsed dye laser
Hair removal–diode laser
Tattoo removal–see chart above
Stretch marks–pulsed dye laser

chapter fifteen

Better Your Body Parts

*You, yourself, as much as anybody in the entire universe,
deserves your love and affection.*

—BUDDHA

IN THE LAST 20 YEARS, THE BABY BOOM HAS TRULY COME INTO ITS OWN. According to the latest figures from the U.S. Census Bureau (1990 census), those aged 50 and over comprise the fastest-growing age group. People, especially women, are living longer than ever before in history, and as one woman recently said, "We are not giving up the fight to look our best." Women feel they are entitled to look as good as possible, as long as possible.

To fight age—and ageism, which results in job loss, rejection on the dating scene, divorce, and untold mental and emotional stress—men and women are dyeing their hair, zapping their wrinkles, dieting, exercising, and signing up for cosmetic surgery procedures. In fact, according to the Plastic Surgery Information Service since 1992 there has been a growing increase in the number of cosmetic surgery procedures performed each year. For example, liposuction rose in excess of 215 percent during that period. Eyelid surgery (blepharoplasty) increased 89 percent. Refusing to give in to wrinkles, sags, and spreading middles, both men and women are seeking cosmetic surgery in record numbers.

Once considered an option only for movie stars, cosmetic surgery is accessible to virtually anyone today. With the help of loans or payment plans, people are seeking out procedures that cost anywhere from several hundred dollars, for example, for collagen injections, to nearly $20,000 for a procedure that combines liposuction with a tummy tuck.

Because laser surgery and facial resurfacing are relatively new, complete figures are not yet available on their huge growth within the industry. One thing you can be certain of: with the world's focus on technology and products that fight aging, you will hear announcements of new information and procedures in the media daily. Stocks of biotech companies are on the rise, as huge corporations strive to find the next formulation or laser to halt the effects of aging.

According to the American Academy of Cosmetic Surgery, the top 10 cosmetic procedures performed in the United States in 1996 were as follows:

Chemical Peel	556,277
Sclerotherapy	516,617
Liposuction	292,942
Hair Transplants	244,466
Laser Resurfacing	138,891
Blepharoplasty	110,492
Rhinoplasty	88,108
Breast Augmentation	76,627
Dermabrasion	68,610
Face-lift	48,943

Many people feel uncomfortable, apologetic, or think others will think they are vain for considering cosmetic surgery. They feel that undergoing such procedures goes against the gains we have made as a society toward accepting people for what they are and the way they are. I asked my friend and colleague Dr. Jack Gorman, a psychiatrist, for his help in explaining why I believe patients should not feel at odds with their decision to improve their appearance.

A Psychiatrist's View of Cosmetic Surgery

By Jack M. Gorman, M.D., Professor of Psychiatry at Columbia University, New York

Even though psychiatrists are generally charged with the responsibility of helping people change, it is also generally assumed that we must always help them to feel happy with their physical appearance. According to that viewpoint, a key role of psychiatric treatment is helping the patient make changes in his or her behavior, mood, and personality, but not in the way they look. In fact, many people who are dissatisfied with the way they look and want a change are sent to psychiatrists for an evaluation and treatment. For the record, I believe that while it is true that some psychiatric disorders are characterized by an abnormal dissatisfaction with some aspect of physical appearance, there is nothing abnormal about wanting to look as good as possible.

Setting aside for the moment political arguments about societal pressure, there is no question that physical appearance influences the quality of an individual's social life and professional accomplishment. Statistics bear out the fact that attractive people receive preferential treatment in many spheres of life. Although this may be morally reprehensible, and we may argue that the proper solution probably is to outlaw discrimination on the basis of physical characteristics, for the individual bothered by some aspect of personal appearance, the call to political arms brings less than satisfaction. For that reason, I believe that as long as society favors physically attractive people and as long as we have safe technology for improving appearance, psychiatrists should never take the position that cosmetic surgery represents a "neurotic" or psychiatrically abnormal attempt to change a personal characteristic. Instead, in most cases, I completely support patients who express a desire to have cosmetic surgery.

To be sure, there are exceptions. A few psychiatric illnesses may involve a misperception of physical appearance. Body dysmorphic disorder, for example, is a condition in which a patient develops a preoccupation with an imagined or greatly exaggerated physical defect. Patients with schizophrenia occasionally develop delusional ideas about their appearance. Patients with anorexia nervosa believe they are fat, even as their weight dips below medically safe levels. Clearly, cosmetic surgery is not appropriate for any of these people, and instead, they require psychiatric treatment. In addition, some people without a psychiatric illness hold an unrealistic idea about the benefits of cosmetic surgery. Such men and women may fantasize that correction of a physical defect, whether real or exaggerated in their minds, will make an enormous difference in their lives. In those cases, if surgery is actually performed, these men and women usually end up disappointed when their lives don't change overnight.

However, in my experience, most people seeking cosmetic surgery realistically believe that they will feel a bit better about themselves and develop a little more self-confidence if they fix an aspect of their physical appearance that bothers them. These individuals, which comprise the majority of people, in my opinion, understand that surgery will not make them the most popular person in school, an instant movie star, or the object of desire by every potential sexual partner. Rather, their goal is to relieve a long-standing and bothersome physical characteristic.

Americans, as a rule, do not live lives in which we accept the cards that are dealt to us at birth. Most people are nearsighted, but we still wear corrective lenses and make those lenses as attractive as possible, even sometimes making them invisible as with contact lenses. Many of us try to alter our appearance by dieting and exercise. These are widely considered positive and healthy actions, yet they still represent efforts to alter the natural state of our physical existence. As long as expectations are realistic, cosmetic surgery seems to me to be part and parcel of the same concept—the important role in our lives of looking (and feeling) good.

When to Go to a Dermatologist Versus a Plastic Surgeon

This is a difficult question to answer fully. Many dermatologists and plastic surgeons, as well as doctors in other areas of specialty, perform cosmetic surgery procedures today. The key to any successful surgery—whether liposuction, face-lift, or laser resurfacing—is to select a physician who has a great deal of experience performing the procedure in which you are interested.

Ask the doctor you are considering the following questions:

"How long have you been doing this procedure?"
"How many of these procedures have you done?"
"What are your credentials?" (Check whether he or she is a board-certified dermatologist or other appropriately trained surgeon.)
"Can I see before and after pictures?"
"Can I speak with your patients?"
"What results can I expect?"
"How long is the recuperation period?"
"What are the risks?"
"Where is the surgery usually performed?"
"What is the worst complication you (the doctor) have ever had?"

Liposuction

For many years, liposuction remained mainly the domain of plastic surgeons. That all changed in 1985 when a dermatologist by the name of Jeffrey Klein, M.D., invented what is now known as tumescent liposuction. With tumescent liposuction (today considered the gold standard of liposuction), a solution composed of saline (salt water), a small amount of lidocaine for anesthesia, and epinephrine (adrenaline) is instilled into the fat while you are awake (local anesthesia). The lidocaine numbs the fat, eliminating the need for general anesthesia. The epinephrine in the solution constricts the blood vessels, which dramatically reduces bleeding. This solution also softens the fat so that it can easily be extracted.

In addition, the saline solution also acts as a fluid replacement, being partly reabsorbed into the body, keeping the patient hydrated, even while much of the saline is suctioned back out with the fat. Because tumescent liposuction was invented by a dermatologist, many dermatologists perform this procedure as well as or better than some plastic surgeons do.

Tumescent liposuction also has now made it possible to extract fat from certain body areas that previously were considered off-limits for liposuction. In the past, for example, the arms, ankles, and calves were considered difficult to liposuction and/or prone to significant risks or complications. The use of tumescent liposuction in conjunction with newer, thinner cannulas now allows these areas to be done with terrific results. (Cannulas are the thin metal rods that are used to suction the fat.)

Choosing the Right Procedure

As Dr. Gorman aptly put it, looks do matter. Are you ready to make a real difference in your looks? If so, you can get rid of unwanted fat, from lovehandles to thunder thighs, puffy tummies, saggy underarms, and even jowls, by getting liposuction. But before you make that appointment, let's go over the facts behind this popular procedure and then I'll give you the latest word on eye jobs and other cosmetic surgeries, even hair transplants. Plus, I'll show you how to test your tolerance for these procedures.

Chin, Neck, and Jowls

The chin, neck, and jowl areas can respond beautifully to liposuction. For many, it is a wonderful alternative to a neck- or face-lift.

A common misconception about liposuction is that the skin will sag after liposuction. In fact, I've found just the opposite to be true: skin tends to retract and redrape nicely once the bulky fat, which has pushed skin out and away from bones and muscles, is removed. So, while liposuction is clearly no replacement for face-lift surgery, suctioning the neck, jowl, and chin can offer a terrific alternative for patients looking for a smaller outpatient procedure, performed under local anesthesia, with minimal risk and downtime.

Who Does This Procedure: A dermatologist, plastic surgeon, or another kind of physician who is highly experienced in this procedure.

Cost: $3,000 to $5,000

Bra Bulge

Another area for which people commonly request liposuction is the back, including the "bra bulge" region (areas that bulge above and below the bra).

Who Does This Procedure: A dermatologist, plastic surgeon, or other experienced physician.

Cost: $3,000 to $4,000

Arms

Sagging upper arms have long been the bane of the existence of many otherwise fit and trim patients, not just overweight patients. As mentioned before, this area was previously considered inappropriate for liposuction, but now is one of the most popular areas for the procedure.

Who Does This Procedure: A dermatologist, plastic surgeon, or other experienced physician.

Cost: $4,000

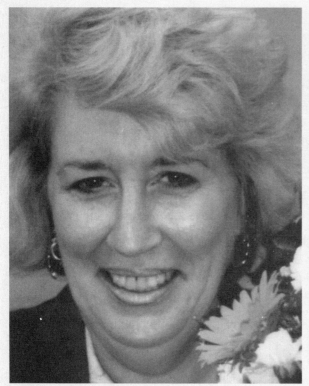

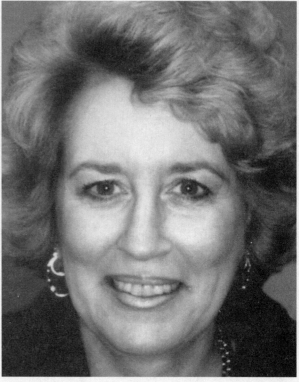

BEFORE: 55-YEAR-OLD WOMAN BEFORE LIPOSUCTION OF THE NECK.

AFTER: PATIENT THREE MONTHS AFTER LIPOSUCTION OF THE NECK. NOTE EXCELLENT SKIN RETRACTION AND WONDERFUL JAWLINE DEFINITION.

Name: DC
Age: 55

PROBLEM:	She wanted to look younger. Although she is not overweight, she looked heavy and matronly, because she had extra flesh around her neck.
WHAT SHE WANTED:	A surgical procedure, since she felt her daily regimen of creams wasn't getting good enough results. She considered a total face-lift, a blepharoplasty (eye job), and/or laser resurfacing.
HER CONCERNS:	She was nervous about having plastic surgery.
DOCTOR'S ADVICE:	I suggested that liposuction of the neck would give her the most subtle, yet best, results.
WHAT SHE HAD DONE:	Liposuction of the neck.
HER REACTION:	"Everyone has been telling me how good I look and wants to know what's different, but no one can figure it out! They think I lost weight (I wish) or got a new haircut."

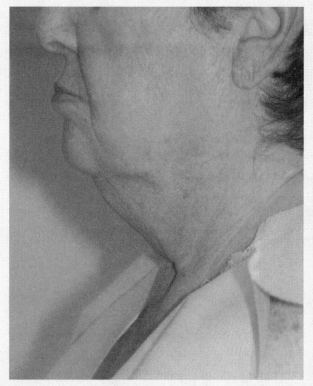

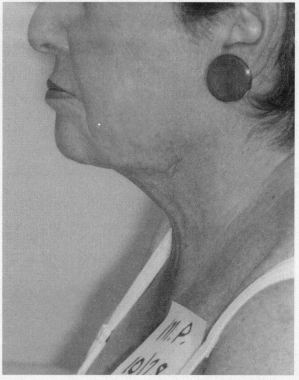

BEFORE: 68-YEAR-OLD WOMAN BEFORE LIPOSUCTION OF THE NECK.

AFTER: PATIENT THREE MONTHS AFTER PROCEDURE. NOTE BEAUTIFUL JAWLINE DEFINITION.

Name: MP
Age: 68

PROBLEM: A heavy neck, which added years to her appearance.
WHAT SHE WANTED: Neck liposuction.
HER CONCERNS: Would the skin be smooth after, or should she have a
                     neck- lift (surgery)?
DOCTOR'S ADVICE: Once the fat in that area is removed, the skin will retract and
                     lie flat, and surgery would be unnecessary.
WHAT SHE HAD DONE: Neck liposuction.
HER REACTION: She was so happy and appreciative, she gave us a beautiful
                     piece of sculpture that she had made herself. I proudly dis-
                     play it in my office.

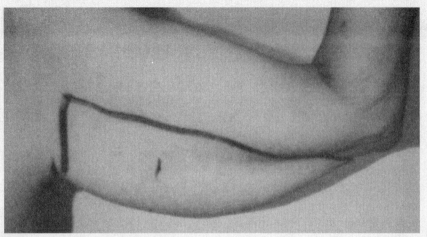

BEFORE: 55-YEAR-OLD WOMAN BEFORE LIPOSUCTION OF THE ARMS.

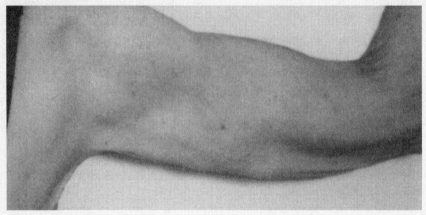

AFTER: PATIENT SIX MONTHS AFTER PROCEDURE. NOTE EXCELLENT SKIN RETRACTION AND MUSCLE DEFINITION NOW VISIBLE SINCE REMOVAL OF EXCESS FAT.

Name: BF
Age: 55

PROBLEM:	Years of weight gain and yo-yo dieting had left fat and sagging skin under her arms.
WHAT SHE WANTED:	Trimmer, firmer upper arms.
HER CONCERNS:	She thought liposuction could not improve the sagging skin.
DOCTOR'S ADVICE:	It certainly would!
WHAT SHE HAD DONE:	Liposuction of the arms.
HER REACTION:	"I am Dr. Bank's biggest cheerleader! I am so happy with how I look now, and I always tell him to have any nervous patients give me a call!"

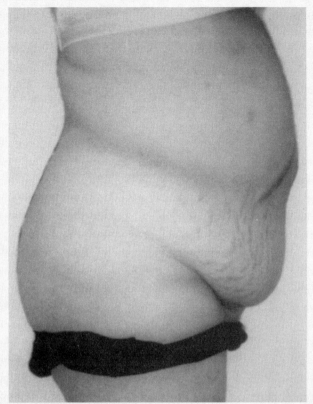 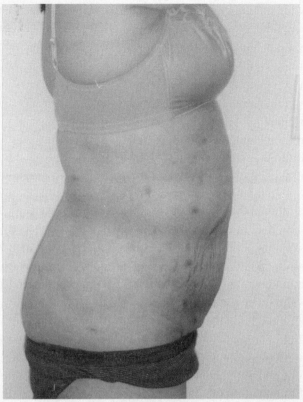

BEFORE: 43-YEAR-OLD WOMAN BEFORE LIPOSUCTION OF THE ABDOMEN, WAIST AND HIPS.

AFTER: PATIENT SIX MONTHS FOLLOWING LIPOSUCTION. NOTE EXCELLENT SKIN RETRACTION.

Name: LK
Age: 43

PROBLEM:	She was a large woman (at 200 pounds), but most of her weight was concentrated in her middle, with a stomach that doubled over.
WHAT SHE WANTED:	To reduce the size of her abdomen.
HER CONCERNS:	She worried that liposuction would leave the skin on her stomach too loose and that she needed a tummy tuck instead.
DOCTOR'S ADVICE:	Contrary to popular belief, liposuction would work wonderfully in this area, because the skin does retract.
WHAT SHE HAD DONE:	Liposuction to remove fat from the upper and lower abdomen, the waist, and the hips.
HER REACTION:	Five days after the operation, she felt and looked great. Six months later, she looked and felt like a new woman. She and her husband are thrilled!

Stomach

Many patients think that if they get their stomach liposuctioned, the "extra" skin covering the suctioned area will then sag or "hang." They convince themselves that they'd be better off getting a tummy tuck instead. This is far from the truth. Many patients, especially if they are younger than 45, get wonderful results with liposuction of the abdomen because after the bulky fat is removed, the skin has a natural tendency to redrape and retract. Young patients who have good skin tone and aren't tremendously overweight will usually find the results they are looking for with liposuction. Even patients in the 45 and older category who are looking to simply debulk the areas will find wonderful results from liposuction. For people who have experienced significant stretching and distension of the stomach skin and muscle (and who may want to wear a bikini in the future), an abdominoplasty, or tummy tuck (more frequently performed by plastic surgeons), may be the procedure of choice.

Who Does This Procedure: A dermatologist, plastic surgeon, or other experienced physician.

Cost: $4,000 to $6,000

Chest

This is another area that can respond well to liposuction. Liposuction on male breasts (gynecomastia) has shown extremely nice results. One exciting new area is breast reduction by liposuction alone. This procedure certainly beats the cost, emotional as well as financial, of breast reduction by plastic surgery, which is a very involved procedure that sometimes leaves unsightly scars.

Who Does This Procedure: A dermatologist, plastic surgeon, or other experienced physician.

Cost: $3,000 to $5,000

Waist

The waist responds tremendously to liposuction, because it tends to drape and retract magnificently after the fat has been removed.

Who Does This Procedure: A dermatologist, plastic surgeon, or other experienced physician.

Cost: $3,000 to $5,000

Hips

Chunky hips are best slimmed down by liposuction.

Who Does This Procedure: A dermatologist, plastic surgeon, or other experienced physician.

Cost: $3,000 to $5,000

Buttocks

The buttocks is a popular area to have liposuctioned. Again, you need someone skillful who can sculpt the buttocks into a pleasing shape. If a doctor is overly aggressive, liposuctioning of the buttocks can lead to sagging, drooping, or even flattened buttocks. If the procedure is performed well and properly, this area lends itself to good results.

Who Does This Procedure: A dermatologist, plastic surgeon, or other experienced physician.

Cost: $3,000 to $5,000

Thighs

Areas of the thighs that respond well to liposuction include the outer thigh, or "saddlebag" area, as well as both the upper and lower inner thigh.

Outer Thigh

Saddlebags (outer thighs) respond beautifully to liposuction because these areas are especially resistant to molding through diet and exercise. Some interesting new studies suggest that this area may contain a deeper layer of fat that is biologically different from the fat just under the skin. This deep, thick fat causes the bulging saddlebags and is extremely difficult to reduce with diet and exercise.

Upper and Lower Thighs

The upper and lower inner thighs is another area that was previously considered a potential problem spot for liposuction. Again, the doctor's experience in liposuctioning this particular region plays a critical part in a successful outcome. In addition, it is important for the physician to place the patient in the proper position during the procedure, so that the muscle, skin, and fat are aligned to match the patient's anatomy when he or she is standing upright. In a number of cases, patients were suctioned in less-than-optimal positions, leading to some divots, or lines or waviness, which later I have been asked to correct in my practice.

Who Does These Procedures: A dermatologist, plastic surgeon, or other experienced physician.

Cost: $4,000 to $6,000

Knees

This is another area that is particularly bothersome to many women, and is hard to reduce even with diet and exercise, but responds beautifully to liposuction.

Who Does This Procedure: A dermatologist, plastic surgeon or, other experienced physician.

Cost: $3,000

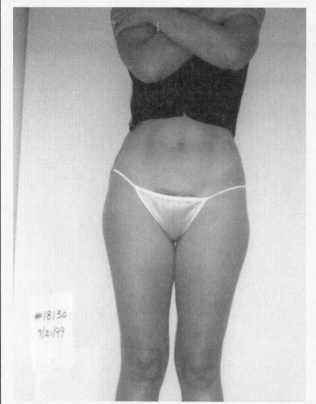

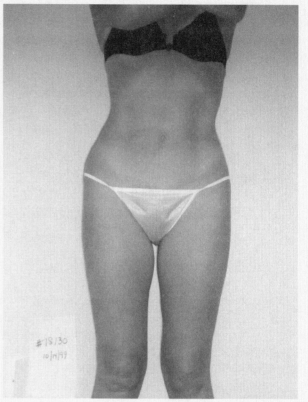

BEFORE: 46-YEAR-OLD WOMAN BEFORE LIPOSUCTION OF THE OUTER THIGHS.

AFTER: NOTE EXCELLENT CONTOUR IMPROVEMENT.

Name: WC
Age: 46

PROBLEM:	Protruding outer thighs, despite years as a dancer and avid exercise.
WHAT SHE WANTED:	Liposuction.
HER CONCERNS:	She feared it would be painful.
DOCTOR'S ADVICE:	Except for the tiny injection to numb the incision point, not much about liposuction is really painful.
WHAT SHE HAD DONE:	Liposuction of the outer thighs.
HER REACTION:	She is thrilled to have dropped several clothing sizes. Finally, she has achieved the silhouette she has worked for all of her life.

Calves and Ankles

Again, as mentioned before, these areas were not considered optimal areas for liposuction, but advances in the procedure have made it very possible to obtain good results.

Who Does This Procedure: A dermatologist, plastic surgeon, or other experienced physician.

Cost: $4,000

When Fat Isn't the Problem…

Liposuction is an ideal option for creating a new silhouette, slimming down a problem area, and correcting a problem of excess fat. Here is the rundown on options for appearance enhancement of other areas of the body.

Eyes

When people speak to each other, they most often focus on each other's eyes and face, and a youthful impression there carries over to the impression of the person as a whole. Any kind of rejuvenating procedure done around the eyes usually produces dramatic results. Patients often come in to see me convinced that lasers are the magic tools for solving all of their problems. Unfortunately, that is not the case. By the same token, other patients come in thinking that a blepharoplasty, or "eye job," will erase all their eye lines; that, too, isn't always true.

When it comes to cosmetic procedures for the eyes, here's what does work:

Sagging Skin Around the Eyes: If the predominant problem is excess sagging skin, especially of the upper or lower eyelids, or if the lower eyelid area bulges, then the best procedure is blepharoplasty. This and other plastic surgery procedures are discussed fully in Chapter 16.

Sun Damage and Wrinkles Around Eyes: If you want to smooth out the skin either under your eyes or around the crow's-feet area that is lined or wrinkled from sun exposure, then you need Botox injections, some type of resurfacing procedure, or a combination of both. Resurfacing can be done with either laser resurfacing (Erbium or carbon dioxide) or with dermabrasion or chemical peels. Laser resurfacing is more commonly performed by dermatologists–see Chapter 14 for more information on all lasers. Overactivity of the muscle in this part of the face causes the majority of wrinkling in the crow's-feet area. The Botox relaxes the overactive muscles, reducing the action that causes the wrinkling. This is why Botox works so well in conjunction with laser resurfacing of the eyes; the Botox relaxes the underlying muscles while the laser smooths the overlying skin. (See Chapter 9 for a complete discussion about Botox.)

Nose Surgery

Reshaping a nose, either for cosmetic reasons or after an accident, is best left to a plastic surgeon or ENT (ear, nose, and throat specialist). This procedure, called rhinoplasty (or nose job), is discussed in Chapter 16.

Lip and Mouth Lines

The lips and mouth can be treated with a number of different enhancement or augmentation procedures. These treatment options include using filler substances, such as collagen, fat injections, and Gore-Tex (see Chapter 9 for a complete description of these procedures), and/or laser resurfacing (see Chapter 14 to read all about laser procedures). Again, as with the eye area, one treatment addresses the underlying "problem" while the laser treats the surface of the skin.

Who Does This Procedure: A dermatologist, plastic surgeon, or other experienced physician.

Hair Transplants

Many men and women undergo hair transplantation procedures to fill in their bald spots and correct a receding hairline. This involves surgically removing hair from one part of the scalp and moving (transplanting) it to the bald or thinning areas. If you decide you want the procedure, you need to consider two things: the qualifications of the doctor and the cause of the balding. I don't think I need to explain about the importance of choosing the right doctor, but it is wise to determine the cause of the hair loss to ensure that it is caused by genetics and is not a symptom of a medical problem. This is especially true for women, who can experience genetic hair loss but may also be affected by hormone imbalances, thyroid problems, responses to medications, anemia (iron deficiency), and lupus (an autoimmune disease). It is prudent to get a medical evaluation of the hair loss before undergoing hair transplant surgery.

Who Does This Procedure: Most often dermatologists, although also plastic surgeons.

Cost: $3,000 to $10,000, depending on the number of hairs transplanted

Leg Veins

When it comes to taking care of their leg veins, many patients start with a visit to a vascular surgeon, who then refers them to a dermatologist for sclerotherapy. Sclerotherapy, or leg vein injections, is a highly effective way to remove spider veins as well as smaller varicose veins. This procedure, which has been around for several decades, consists of a series of three or four treatments, with about four weeks between each treatment. The patient is instructed to wear compression stockings immediately after the procedure to compress the treated blood vessels so that they will seal up and die.

Who Does This Procedure: Most dermatologists receive sclerotherapy training as part of their education and certification programs. Some plastic surgeons may perform the procedure, but you should always ask how many they have done.

Cost: $350 per session

Test Your Tolerance Level

When it comes to cosmetic surgery, whether liposuction, a peel, microdermabrasion, laser surgery, or Botox injections, different people have different levels of tolerance. A treatment one person might consider an absolute must that is well worth the accompanying discomfort, another person might need to think hard about doing, while yet another person would never even entertain the thought. People's reasons for being receptive or unreceptive to cosmetic procedures also vary. Some folks will put up with discomfort because they desire the end result. Others won't even consider the treatment, even though they may desire the same result, because they are afraid they won't be able to handle the discomfort. Also, some patients view the procedures as being impractical, because they can't or won't make time in their schedules for adequate downtime or recovery.

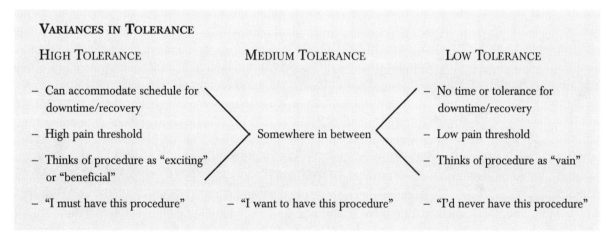

VARIANCES IN TOLERANCE

HIGH TOLERANCE	MEDIUM TOLERANCE	LOW TOLERANCE
– Can accommodate schedule for downtime/recovery		– No time or tolerance for downtime/recovery
– High pain threshold	Somewhere in between	– Low pain threshold
– Thinks of procedure as "exciting" or "beneficial"		– Thinks of procedure as "vain"
– "I must have this procedure"	– "I want to have this procedure"	– "I'd never have this procedure"

The difference between the high, medium, and low tolerance levels also relates to a patient's concept of "aging gracefully."

Some view aging as the natural progression of the effects of time and personal habits (like smoking or sun exposure) on the skin and the body. Others say the "graceful" part comes as a result of fighting time and gravity with all available means. You must determine for yourself how you feel about certain procedures in order for your expectations and the success of the procedure to be in sync.

chapter sixteen

A Plastic Surgery Primer

*The future belongs to those who believe
in the beauty of their dreams.*
—ELEANOR ROOSEVELT

HERE, FOR YOUR READING PLEASURE, ARE DESCRIPTIONS OF THE MOST COMMON plastic surgery procedures.

Breast Augmentation (Augmentation Mammaplasty)

What It Is: A safe, effective surgical procedure designed to improve the contour of a woman's body by implanting specially designed materials beneath the breast or chest-wall muscles.

Before Surgery: Prior to surgery, a complete medical history is taken to evaluate the general health of the patient. An examination of the breasts is also made to determine the most effective surgical approach. The physician describes the type of anesthesia to be used, the procedure, what results might realistically be expected, and the possible risks and complications. Mammograms or X-rays and photographs may be taken as well.

Procedure: A breast augmentation is usually performed in a hospital or an outpatient surgical setting under general anesthesia. The physician may choose from a variety of surgical procedures, depending on the nature and extent of changes desired. An incision is made in the lower portion of the breast near the chest wall or sometimes near the armpit. The breast tissue is raised to create a pocket either under the breast tissue or beneath the chest-wall muscle, and the implant is inserted. After the implant is securely in place, small sutures are used to close the incision.

Pain Quotient: Pain connected with the procedure is minimal to moderate and is controlled with oral medication.

After Surgery: The patient wears either bandages or a special garment immediately after surgery. These are usually replaced in a few days with a surgical bra, which is worn for several weeks. Antibiotics may be prescribed to prevent infection. Instructions for the day of surgery include bed rest and limited activities. Sutures are removed in about five to seven days. Swelling and discoloration disappear in a few days, and scars fade significantly with time.

Cost: $4,000 to $5,000

Breast Lift (Mastopexy)

What It Is: A breast lift, or mastopexy, can correct sagging or loose breasts resulting from pregnancy, weight loss, or natural aging. This procedure is designed to elevate and reshape the breast. Mastopexy is often performed in conjunction with surgery designed to enlarge the breasts.

Before Surgery: Prior to surgery, a complete medical history is taken to evaluate the general health of the patient. An examination of the breasts also is made to determine the most effective surgical approach. The physician describes the type of anesthesia to be used, the procedure, what results might realistically be expected, and possible risks and complications. Mammograms or X-rays and photographs may be taken before surgery.

Procedure: A breast lift is usually performed in a hospital or outpatient surgical facility. The physician may choose from a variety of procedures, depending on the nature and extent of changes desired. Usually under a general anesthesia, incisions are made, excess skin is removed, and underlying tissue is then repositioned into a new, higher location. The skin is sutured together to reshape the breast.

Pain Quotient: Minimal to moderate, which is controlled with oral medication.

After Surgery: Following surgery, the patient wears either bandages or a special garment. This is usually replaced with a surgical bra, which is worn for several weeks. The physician determines when the patient can resume normal activities; however, the patient must avoid strenuous exercise and overhead lifting for several weeks. Sutures are removed in about seven to 10 days, and scars will fade significantly in time.

Cost: $3,500 to $4,500

Breast Reduction (Reduction Mammaplasty)

What It Is: Breast reduction, or reduction mammaplasty, is designed to improve the body contour and to reduce the pain and discomfort of women with large, sagging, or uneven breasts.

Before Surgery: Prior to surgery, a complete medical history is taken to evaluate the general health of the patient. The breasts are examined to determine the most effective surgical approach. The physician describes the type of anesthesia to be used, the procedure, what results might realistically be expected, and possible risks and complications. Mammograms or X-rays and photographs may be taken. Preoperative instructions often include the elimination of certain drugs containing aspirin for several weeks before surgery to minimize the possibility of excess bleeding.

Procedure: A breast reduction is usually performed in a hospital or outpatient surgical setting usually with a general anesthesia. The physician may choose from a variety of surgical procedures, depending on the nature and extent of changes desired. Incisions are made; excess fat, tissue, and skin are removed; and the incision is then sutured.

Pain Quotient: Pain connected with the procedure is minimal to moderate and is controlled with oral medication. Instructions for the day of surgery include bed rest with limited activities.

After Surgery: Following surgery, the patient wears either bandages or a special garment. These are usually replaced in a few days with a surgical bra, which is worn for several weeks. The physician determines when the patient can resume normal activities; however, the patient must avoid strenuous exercise and overhead lifting for several weeks. Sutures are removed in about seven days. Swelling and discoloration disappear in a few days, and scars fade significantly with time.

Cost: $6,000 to $7,000

Cheek Implant (Malar Augmentation)

What It Is: Cheek implants, or malar augmentation, can give a person the high cheekbones he or she desires. This surgery can give definition to a face that has a flat contour resulting from underdeveloped cheekbones. It also can benefit people with asymmetries or congenital defects of the face.

Before Surgery: Prior to surgery, a complete medical history is taken to evaluate the general health of the patient. The physician describes to the patient the type of anesthesia to be used, the procedure, what results might realistically be expected, and possible risks and complications.

Procedure: Cheek implants can be performed in a physician's office, an outpatient surgical facility, or a hospital, depending on the physician's and patient's preferences, using a local or general anesthesia. The face is thoroughly cleansed with an antiseptic cleansing agent, after which an incision is made either inside the mouth or immediately below the lower eyelids. The implant is inserted, and tiny sutures are used to close the incisions.

Pain Quotient: Pain connected with the surgery is minimal to moderate and is controlled with oral medication.

After Surgery: Sutures are removed within a week. The patient may experience difficulty chewing for about two weeks as well as tightness or numbness around the treated area for a period of time. Brushing the teeth is often difficult for several days.

Cost: $2,000

Chin Implant (Mentoplasty)

What It Is: Chin implant, or mentoplasty, is a surgical procedure designed to add size to or move forward a receding chin. The best candidate for chin augmentation is the individual with a receding chin and a normal dental bite.

Before Surgery: Prior to surgery, a complete medical history is taken to evaluate the general health of the patient. The physician describes the type of anesthesia to be used, the procedure, what results might realistically be expected, and possible risks and complications.

Procedure: The surgery can be done in a physician's office, an outpatient surgical facility, or a hospital, depending on the physician's and patient's preferences, using a local or general anesthesia. Two basic procedures are used in mentoplasty: one involves moving the chin bone forward, and the other involves inserting a plastic chin implant. In both procedures, incisions are made under the chin or in the mouth and the bone is cut; the bone is then either moved or the implant is inserted. Sutures are used to close the incision, and pressure bandages are applied.

Pain Quotient: Pain connected with the surgery is minimal to moderate and is controlled with oral medication.

After Surgery: The bandages are usually removed within a week. Patients are up and moving around the day of surgery; however, patients must avoid strenuous activities for some time. The physician determines when normal activities can be resumed, based on the extent of surgery and the patient's healing process. The patient may experience difficulty chewing for 10 days to two weeks as well as numbness around the treatment area.

Cost: $2,000

Ear Surgery (Otoplasty)

What It Is: Otoplasty, sometimes described as "pinning" the ears, is designed to change the shape and contour of an ear. It may be performed on anyone over the age of five or six years.

Before surgery: Prior to surgery, a medical history is taken to evaluate the general health of the patient. The physician and patient, or adult family member (for example, when the patient is a minor), discuss how the ears should look and what can realistically be expected. The type of anesthesia to be used, the procedure, and possible risks and complications are also discussed.

Procedure: Otoplasty can be done under general anesthesia with the patient asleep or under local anesthesia with the area numbed and the patient remaining awake. A basic procedure involves an incision being made at the back of the ear to expose the cartilage. The cartilage is reshaped, the incisions are closed with small sutures, and the ears are covered with bandages.

Pain Quotient: Pain connected with the surgery is minimal to moderate and is controlled with oral medication.

After Surgery: Bandages are removed within a few days but may be replaced with a lighter head dressing. Bruising around the area occurs but fades within a few weeks. Scars from the incisions fade significantly in time and are usually inconspicuous, because the incisions are made within the creases of the ears.

Cost: $2,000 to $3,000

Surgery of the Eyes (Blepharoplasty), Brow, and Forehead Lift

What It Is: Blepharoplasty, or eyelid surgery, can correct sagging eyelids, pouches beneath the eyes, and excess folds around the eyes. This surgical procedure involves the removal of excess skin and fat on upper and lower eyelids, resulting in a smoother, more youthful appearance. Brow and forehead lifts are designed to raise eyebrows and to reduce ridges and furrows on the forehead.

Before Surgery: Prior to surgery, a complete medical history is taken to evaluate the general health of the patient. The amount, distribution, and type of excess skin to be removed are carefully noted. The physician describes the anesthesia to be used, the procedure, what results might realistically be expected, and possible risks and complications

Procedure: Blepharoplasty can be performed under general anesthesia with the patient asleep or under local anesthesia with the area numbed and the patient remaining awake. Incisions are made following natural lines and creases. Excess fat and skin are then removed from the underlying compartments. The amount of fat excised is determined by the degree of protrusion of fat when pressure is gently applied to the area. Small sutures are used to close the incision, and special ointments and dressing may be applied.

For a brow or forehead lift, the incision is hidden in the hairline, the forehead and brows are elevated and excess skin is removed, and the incision is sutured.

Pain Quotient: Pain connected with the surgery is minimal to moderate and is controlled with oral medication.

After Surgery: Sutures are removed within a week. Some swelling and bruising occur but subside in a few days. The physician determines when normal activities can be resumed; however, the patient must avoid strenuous exercise for several weeks following surgery.

Cost: $4,000 to $5,000

Face-lift (Rhytidectomy)

What It Is: A face-lift, or rhytidectomy, is designed to correct sagging skin and prominent skin folds, particularly around the chin, along the jaw line, and on the neck. This procedure involves the tightening of facial and neck skin and muscles and the removal of excess skin, resulting in a more youthful appearance. A face-lift can be performed any time after signs of aging appear.

Before Surgery: Prior to surgery, a medical history is taken to evaluate the general health of the patient. The physician and patient discuss together how the face should look and what results can realistically be expected. The goal of the surgery is to produce a pleasing natural appearance. Photographs are taken before and after surgery to determine the amount of improvement. The type of anesthesia to be used, the procedure, and possible risks and complications are also discussed by the physician and patient.

Procedure: The surgery can be performed in a physician's office, an outpatient surgical facility, or a hospital, depending on the physician's and patient's preference. It can be done under general anesthesia with the patient asleep or under local anesthesia with the area numbed and the patient remaining awake. Premedication is usually administered to relax the patient. In the basic procedure, incisions are made along the hairline at the temple, in front of the ear, then around the earlobe and behind the ear, ending in the hair of the scalp. Loose skin, connective tissue, and sagging muscles are tightened, and tiny sutures are used to close the incisions.

Pain Quotient: Pain connected with the surgery is minimal to moderate and is controlled with oral medication.

After Surgery: Loose bandages are applied to the area and removed within a few days. The surgeon determines when to remove sutures. Scars from the incisions fade significantly with time and are usually inconspicuous, because they are made within natural creases. Swelling and discoloration disappear in a week or two. The patient may experience a tightness or numbness at the treated area for a while. For several weeks after surgery, patients should avoid the sun as much as possible and wear sunscreen when outside. Healing is gradual, and final results may not be apparent for several weeks. In most cases, a single procedure achieves the desired results.

Cost: $6,000 to $7,000

Nose Surgery (Rhinoplasty)

What It Is: Nasal reconstruction, or rhinoplasty, was one of the first cosmetic procedures ever developed, and it is among the most frequently performed cosmetic surgeries today. Rhinoplasty is a surgical procedure in which deformities of the nose are corrected by removing, rearranging, or reshaping bone or cartilage. Patients typically desire this surgery to improve the shape of their noses. Both profile and frontal face views can be altered through rhinoplasty.

Before Surgery: Prior to surgery, a medical history is taken to evaluate the general health of the patient. The physician and patient discuss together how the nose should look in relation to the patient's other facial features. It is important for the patient to understand that the goal of the surgery is not to achieve perfection but rather to improve the appearance. The type of anesthesia to be used, the procedure, and possible risks and complications are also discussed.

Procedure: Rhinoplasty can be done under general anesthesia with the patient asleep or under local anesthesia with the area numbed and the patient remaining awake. The procedure is determined by the type of correction to be made. In most cases involving a reduction in size or shape of the nose, the removal of a hump, or the improvement of an angle, incisions are made inside the nose. Working through these incisions, the physician is able to reshape the nose by reworking the bone and cartilage.

Pain Quotient: Pain connected with the surgery is minimal to moderate and is controlled with oral medication.

After Surgery: Following surgery, a lightweight splint is applied to maintain the new shape of the nose; the splint is usually removed within a week. Nasal pads may be inserted at the time of surgery to protect the septum. This packing is removed within a day or two. Swelling and bruising around the treated areas diminish and may be helped with cold compresses. During the healing process, great care must be taken to protect the nose from injury. Although patients are usually up and around a day or two after the procedure, patients should avoid strenuous exercise, particularly that which might elevate blood pressure, for a while.

Cost: $3,000 to $4,000

Tummy Tuck (Abdominoplasty)

What It Is: An abdominoplasty, or tummy tuck (which is not a substitute for weight loss), improves the contour of the body by flattening and narrowing the abdomen. The best candidate for the surgery is a person of normal weight who has weak abdominal muscles and excess skin and fat. This condition does not respond well to diet or exercise, because the skin and underlying muscles have been stretched, often due to prior weight gain or pregnancy.

Before Surgery: Prior to surgery, a complete medical history is taken to evaluate the general health of the patient. The physician and patient discuss together what can realistically be expected. Photographs may be taken before and after surgery to evaluate the amount of improvement. The type of anesthesia to be used, the procedure, and possible risks and complications are also discussed.

Procedure: Abdominoplasty is usually performed in a hospital setting under general anesthesia. Incisions are often made along the lower abdomen.

The skin is lifted, and weak abdominal muscles are sutured to tighten those that are loose or stretched out. The skin is then lowered over the abdomen, and excess skin and fat are removed. The incisions are closed, and often drains are inserted to eliminate fluid buildup. Elastic bandages are then applied to the area.

Pain Quotient: Pain is moderate and can be controlled by oral medication.

After Surgery: Sutures are removed approximately one week after surgery, and bandages are applied. The bandages are later replaced with an abdominal support garment that is worn for several weeks. During this time, patients must refrain from heavy lifting, straining, or overactivity. Although patients are usually up and around the day of surgery, the physician decides when normal activities may be resumed.

Cost: $4,000 to $5,000

chapter seventeen

The Cellulite Solution

No pessimist ever discovered the secret of the stars, or sailed to an uncharted land, or opened a new doorway for the human spirit.
—Helen Keller

It is an ugly fact of life for 90 percent of women: cellulite, those unsightly fatty deposits also known as orange-peel skin. More than just ordinary fat, cellulite is a specific combination of fat, waste, and water that forms a bumpy, rippled mass that gets trapped in the fibrous, connective tissue just below the skin's surface. Cellulite appears most commonly on the hips, thighs, and buttocks, but it can show up on the arms, abdomen, and upper back as well. Several factors contribute to cellulite, including diet as well as a sluggish blood and lymphatic circulation, which allows wastes to accumulate. But three contributing agents determine whether you develop cellulite: heredity, estrogen, and fat. If just one of those ingredients is missing, you don't have cellulite, just plain ordinary fat.

It's in Your Genes (and Your Jeans)

You usually inherit cellulite, that is, if your mom has it–and by "it" we mean loose connective tissue, which fat globules pop up through–chances are you do or will too, even if you're thin. As connective tissue weakens with age, the dimpling becomes even more pronounced. If you have thin skin, which is also hereditary, cellulite is even easier to see than it is on thicker skin.

If your mother has cellulite, you've probably inherited her loosely woven connective tissue and poor lymphatic drainage, which leads to bunched-up fat cells. And as you now know, cellulite is more than just fat: It's fat trapped by a network of connective tissue fibers. If the underlying network is loosely woven, the fat bulges through the fibers, causing a "cottage cheese" effect on the skin. As connective tissue weakens with age, the dimpling becomes even more pronounced.

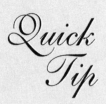

The fibers that extend from the muscle up through the fat and connect to the undersurface of the skin run directly up and down, perpendicularly, at a 90-degree angle, which allows bulging and puckering. In men, the fibers I mentioned run in a crisscross, at a 45-degree angle, so the fat is less likely to bulge up like it does in women.

The "Luck" of the Estrogen

Once women reach puberty, the body's ovaries begin to produce the hormone estrogen, which helps to store fat in the hips, thighs, and buttocks, in preparation for childbearing. We can also thank estrogen for adding to cellulite's puckered appearance: It makes fat cells sticky, so they bunch together like grapes, contributing to the appearance of cellulite.

Diet Dilemmas

Diet plays only a small role in curbing cellulite, because cellulite is basically a genetic, hormonal, and anatomic problem. Dieting can help, especially if you are overweight, but it definitely won't totally solve the problem. In fact, some anorexic women have cellulite. Some overweight women don't show it at all.

Danielle M. Schupp, a registered dietitian and sports nutritionist at Reebok Sports Club, New York, New York, who also owns a private consulting practice, recommends that you exercise regularly and eat a low-fat diet in which 20 to 25 percent of your daily intake of calories comes from fat.

Ms. Schupp suggests following the basic food pyramid discussed in Chapter 8. The example, below, can serve as a quick guide. You should also realize that individual servings and calorie intake will vary. A registered dietitian can provide you with customized diet based on your individual weight goals and level of physical activity.

Sample Plan—1500 Calorie Plan

Breakfast:	1 cup whole grain cereal (5 grams of fiber per serving) with 1 cup skim or low-fat soy milk
	1 Tbs. crushed nuts
	1 small banana
Lunch:	3 ounces turkey on two slices whole grain bread
	Lettuce and tomato and mustard or low-fat mayonnaise
	Salad (include red, green, yellow vegetables) with 2 Tbs. vinaigrette dressing
Snack:	1 cup nonfat yogurt
	1 cup cantaloupe

Dinner: 4 ounces grilled fish, chicken, or lean red meat
           1 small baked sweet potato with one tsp. whipped butter
           1 cup steamed broccoli
Snack: 1 glass skim milk
           1 apple

Serving Guide: 80–100 Calories per Serving

Corn and peas:	1/2 cup
Yam and potato:	1 small potato (3 oz.)
1/2 bagel:	2 oz.
Pasta/grains/rice:	1/2 cup
Pretzels:	3/4 ounce

A diet high in insoluble fiber (wheat bran, fruits, veggies) and with plenty of water and accompanied by lots of physical activity is the best way to achieve a "clean" system. Green tea also can help clean out your system.

Remember: When you reduce the amount of fat in your diet, you reduce the amount of calories you consume. For instance, there are only four calories per gram of carbohydrates and protein, but there are nine calories per gram of fat. So, for every gram of fat you eliminate from your diet, you get double the benefit in terms of weight loss that you would get for every gram of protein or carbohydrates that you eliminate from your diet. But, do not eat less than 20 percent of your calories from fat.

News Worth Swallowing

According to Schupp, as we age, the natural bacterial flora in our large intestine decrease. She suggests eating lacidophilus, found in natural foods such as yogurt (and as a supplement), to assist in digestion. Acidophilus (also found in natural yogurt or supplements) may also help.

Tighten and Tone Up

One way to specifically target the fat under the loose skin is to firm up the muscle under the skin, which will make the skin look tighter and smoother. Fitness expert Joyce L. Vedral, Ph.D., in her cellulite-fighting book *Bottoms Up!* (Warner), uses super sets, doing two exercises one after another quickly, with each exercise hitting a different muscle group, which allows one set of muscles to relax while another set is being worked to exhaustion. This helps to build tone and muscle, which smooths out the appearance of cellulite and makes the skin look firmer. An added benefit of exercise: It helps get your circulation going.

Creams and Potions

Cellulite is a three-dimensional problem that involves the entire fatty layer and extends all the way from under the surface of the skin down to the muscle. Consequently, topically applied creams have little chance of success at busting cellulite. No cream applied to the skin's surface can penetrate completely through the skin, cause the fat cells to detach from each other, improve the lymphatic circulation, and reduce the skin's swelling. If applying lotion seems to bring any improvement at all, it's probably due to massaging or rubbing in the cream, which can lessen the swelling and improve the lymphatic drainage in the area. However, whatever minor, and temporary, improvement you might gain has nothing to do with the active ingredient in the cream, which does nothing at all to cellulite.

Ultrasound

Ultrasound is an interesting concept for combating cellulite. Unfortunately, no benefit in terms of reducing or eliminating or in any way changing the composition of cellulite has ever been derived from zapping it with ultrasound.

Why Liposuction Doesn't Work

Contrary to popular belief, cellulite is not an indication for liposuction. Liposuction is terrific for removing excess deposits of fat or bulges (places where fat cells clump together). That's why it's perfect for love handles, bulges at the thighs, abdomen, hips, upper arms, and other such fat deposits. So, if you need to debulk unwanted fat cells, lipo works. However, if you have a good silhouette (no obvious bumps or lumps) when wearing leggings and a bodysuit, but you still have cellulite, then liposuction won't get rid of the ripples and dimples.

Bottom line: Liposuction can remove excess fat cells, but it cannot affect how they organize themselves or their general structure.

The Newest Discovery: Cellasene (But Hold On!)

Again, put your money back in your pocket and don't waste it on Cellasene, the expensive new herbal anticellulite product from Italy. This is merely a magical-sounding mixture of common supplements, which are touted by the product's manufacturer to increase blood circulation, reduce fluid buildup, and stimulate metabolism. None of the cited studies have been peer-reviewed, and the studies lacked proper controls. Cellasene seems to contain nothing more than several herbs that have no effect on the biology of the human body. Bottom line: save your money.

What Works

Because cellulite is a three-dimensional problem under the skin all the way down to the muscle, and because it has to do with fat cells swelling up and sticking and bunching together, no topical cream is likely to have much effect. Therefore, the only treatment options with any chance of success are those that involve manipulation of the full thickness of the fatty layer.

Deep Tissue Massage

Currently, the only treatment available that has been shown to offer any benefit at all for cellulite is deep tissue massage. This procedure goes by several trade names, including Endermologie, by LPG, and Silhouette, by Luxar. This course of therapy consists of a series of treatments, usually two treatments a week, each lasting about thirty-five minutes, for eight to 10 weeks.

How It Works: A physician or a physician's assistant moves a machine, basically a vacuum with two rollers attached to the end of a hose, across the cellulite-plagued area. The suction action of the machine results in a very deep massage. Supposedly, as the machine massages, the motion "wrings" the extra fluid out of the swollen fat cells and out from between the cells, in the process improving the lymphatic drainage. The effect is to convert the fat from a group of clumped-up, swollen grapes to rows of eggs all neatly stacked in a row, letting the skin lie smoothly on top. In theory, this sounds wonderful. In real life, the results can vary from modest to rather impressive.

Cost: $100 a session; a minimum of 14 sessions performed twice a week for several weeks are recommended.

Drawback: The improvement is temporary. If you decide to undergo the deep massage process, you must commit to a long treatment time (at least fourteen treatments).

Exercise

Exercise can definitely help, but because of the swelling of the fat cells and the matrix of the connecting fibrous bands, exercise alone won't solve the problem. I see many patients who are in excellent shape and condition, including professional athletes, who suffer from cellulite. Others are couch potatoes and have no cellulite. Go figure.

Get Tuff by Tanning

Tanning the area where you have cellulite can make it appear less noticeable. However, the sun causes collagen in the skin to stretch and change, which can actually magnify the look of cellulite. So, as I've said before, nix the sun. A better bet is to apply a self-tanning product. (Try either Neutrogena Sunless Tanning Spray or Physicians Formula Sunless Tanning Lotion.) To self-tan: first, gently rub an exfoliating cream onto the area to rid it of all dead skin cells. Rinse it off in the shower, and dry thoroughly with a towel. Next, apply the self-tanner, using a circular upward motion. Lie on your stomach on a towel as the cream dries.

Did you know that…

A good reason to strength-train: Unless we do it regularly after age 25, we lose up to a half-pound of muscle every year. But if we do strength-train, adding just three pounds of muscle increases our metabolic rate by up to 7 percent (which means we can eat more calories).

chapter eighteen

Dangerous Beauty

Nothing in the world is more dangerous than sincere ignorance and conscientious stupidity.

—Martin Luther King, Jr.

SHOULD YOU DYE YOUR EYELASHES, BUY A PRODUCT THAT SAYS IT WILL ACCELERATE your tan, or try a high-powered bleaching cream you find abroad? Sounds appealing, but according to the Food and Drug Administration (FDA), your answers to all of these scenarios should be a sound "No." Greedy entrepreneurs make millions of dollars every day at consumers' expense, touting their visions of youth through wrinkle remedies, breast-stimulating devices, or hair loss creams. Ultimately, in most cases, the only one who gets creamed is you, the consumer. This chapter provides you with real information on the latest health and beauty fads—and on why they're so bad for you.

Color to Die For

Many women consider dyeing their eyelashes (as well as their hair) a normal part of a beauty routine. But is it safe? "No", says the Food and Drug Administration (FDA), which maintains that hair dyes for eyelashes—both salon and home varieties—can cause serious injuries, even blindness, if washed into the eyes.

At present, no dyes (natural or synthetic) have been approved for lashes or brows. In the 1930s, the FDA banned these types of products after two accidents in which one woman died and another was blinded. Consumers should never dye their eyebrows or eyelashes. An allergic reaction to the dye could prompt swelling, inflammation, and susceptibility to infection in the eye area. These reactions can severely harm the eye and even cause blindness. The FDA prohibits the use of hair dyes and coal-tar dyes for eyebrow and eyelash tinting or dyeing, even in beauty salons and other establishments.

Tanning Accelerators

The FDA has ruled that manufacturers of accelerated tanning products can't make claims to "speed up your natural tanning process and promote deeper, faster tanning," because none of the products have been approved by the FDA as drugs (affecting structure or function of the human body). Some companies have removed such language from their advertisements.

Actually, most tanning accelerators are only moisturizers and do nothing to increase skin's melanin, as they claim. Most also don't contain sunscreen, so they offer no protection against the sun.

Bleaching Creams

Hydroquinone (HQ), an FDA-approved drug, is the active ingredient in bleaching creams, which work by stopping the skin's overproduction of melanin. In 1982, the FDA deemed skin bleaches to be safe and effective for use on age spots, freckles, and hormone-induced dark spots–but not for use as an all-over skin lightener.

Many over-the-counter HQ bleaching products exceed the FDA's 2 percent concentration limit, such as monobenzone, which was taken off the market a number of years ago.

Self-Tanning Pills

It sounds wonderful: Swallow a pill and, boom, you're sporting a deep, dark tan. Don't believe it. Tanning pills are FDA-prohibited and illegal. These internal dye jobs contain synthetic versions of two food colors, beta carotene and canthaxanthin, chemical replicas of substances that occur naturally in certain plants.

Canthaxanthin is approved for coloring some foods and drugs, but the FDA has not okayed it for internal use to tint the human body. After a week or two, the dye accumulates in the skin, and voilà!–you are tan. Unfortunately, over time the body gets such a color overdose that some accumulates in the blood, the skin, fatty tissue, and the liver. This results in severe itching, skin eruptions, nausea, diarrhea, and even night blindness and hepatitis.

In one tragic instance, a 20-year-old woman died of a rare blood disease after taking tanning pills. Although available in Canada and Europe, they remain illegal in America.

Tattoo? Not You!

Although tattoos are all the rage, many states do not regulate the business. The mercurials and sulfurs used in tattooing often cause allergic reactions. The danger of tattoos lies primarily in the possibility of infection due to unsterile equipment. Dirty needles can spread diseases, such as hepatitis and

AIDS. Patients can suffer an allergic reaction to the color dyes. The colors of the tattoo can also "drift" out of the original area, causing a blurry-looking tattoo.

And what if you change your mind after the fact? Removing tattoos is possible, but painful and costly. Also, when you remove a tattoo, it always leaves a mark on the skin. If you must get a tattoo, your best bet is to go to places and people that you know are reputable. The facility you select should supply surgical gloves for practitioners, sterilize all equipment, and use new needles for each customer.

Permanent Makeup

Permanent makeup (such as eyeliner, lipliner or color, and eyebrows) presents the same dangers as tattoos (which they essentially are).

This practice originated from the initial use of pigmentation as a medical treatment to put the color back into areola and nipple areas of the breast after mastectomies. Now, it is being used as a beauty treatment for applying permanent lip and eyelining by many beauty salons. Using disposable needles, pigment that is derived from vegetable products is implanted into the skin at the base of the upper or lower eyelashes. A local anesthetic is often given to relieve pain during the tattooing, which takes from 20 minutes to an hour.

But, points out chemist John Bailey, Ph.D., director of the FDA's colors and cosmetics program, "We can't vouch for the safety of permanent eyelining," because the procedure hasn't undergone any formal safety testing. The FDA is currently considering requiring safety testing for tattooed eyeliner. If such testing finds permanent eyelining unsafe, the FDA could ban the procedure, because it uses colors that are under the agency's jurisdiction.

Cures for Baldness

At this point in time, the only prescription product that has been approved for growing hair on balding men is Propecia. Rogaine (minoxidil) is now available over-the-counter without a prescription.

Breast and Muscle Stimulators

Many muscle stimulators are used legitimately in a medical capacity to increase blood circulation, prevent clots, relax muscle spasms, and rehabilitate muscles after a stroke. However, others are being promoted as having the ability to remove wrinkles, do no-surgery face-lifts, get rid of cellulite, and reduce or increase breast size. Their claims are absolutely unfounded, and the FDA considers the promotion of these devices for those claims to be fraudulent.

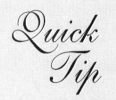

Quick Tip

To keep cosmetic brushes in tip-top condition: Wash them in a delicate fabric wash or baby shampoo. Rinse well and lay the brushes flat to dry.

Bite Your Tongue

According to the American Dental Association, tongue-piercing poses a huge health hazard. The FDA's formal policy statement warns that if you pierce your tongue, you run the risk of hitting a nerve and deadening the tongue. Then, you would have difficulty chewing food for the rest of your life, and you could also lose your sense of taste as well as your ability to speak clearly. Other potential dangers include: scar tissue, infection, allergic reaction, and disease (from tainted needles). Need they say more?

Skin 911

At times, despite your best intentions (and most careful shopping), you end up using or buying a product that brings out some kind of a reaction (and not necessarily a good one). Here's the meaning of these reactions, and a few easy solutions.

You feel tenderness or see swelling: This indicates an inflammation. Try cool milk compresses to reduce the symptoms. If the condition doesn't clear up within three days, see a doctor.

You feel itchy: You are possibly experiencing an allergic reaction to a medication, skin care product, or makeup product. To soothe the itching, apply cold compresses and make an appointment to see a dermatologist. If your eyelids feel scratchy and itchy, you may be reacting to either the latex or nickel in your eyelash curler or even possibly to the formaldehyde in your nail polish. Switching to a formaldehyde-free formula will probably help clear it up. If your hairline or head is itchy, or even red and scaly, you may have an allergic reaction to any of the hair products you are using. Stop using the products (especially if you are using something new) and see your dermatologist.

Common Questions

Q: I wear fake nails and think that I may have a fungal infection, because I haven't taken them off in a year. What should I do?

A: One way to check for a fungus infection is to see whether any brown, yellow, or green gunk appears where the nails attach to the skin. Other signs include thickened nails, gunk under the nails, and yellowed nails. Even if you have none of these symptoms, keeping fake nails on for more than six months without removing them (even if they are not broken or chipped) is looking for trouble. Remove them yourself with a solvent or run to your manicurist. In a worse-case scenario, a dermatologist can remove them as well. If you do have a fungus infection, an antifungal cream may do the trick, or you may need an oral dose of antifungal medicine. In the future, remember to always take time to give your real nails some room to breathe every few months.

Q: Is there any particular beauty workshop or program out there for cancer patients?

A: Yes. The "Look Good...Feel Better" course, available around the country, was developed jointly in 1989 for national use by the Cosmetic, Toiletry, and Fragrance Association (CTFA) Foundation, the National Cosmetology Association, and the American Cancer Society. This program attempts to help patients learn to minimize the side effects of cancer drugs and radiation treatment, which can cause changes in hair, complexion, and nails. The course helps teach cancer patients how to apply makeup, formulate a personalized skin-care routine, and work with wigs, turbans, and scarves. It includes group or one-on-one makeover workshops conducted by specially trained volunteer cosmetologists in hospitals, community centers, and salons. For help locating a "Look Good...Feel Better" program, call the local chapter of the American Cancer Society or 800-395-LOOK.

Q: Can manufacturers simply put their most chemical or caustic ingredients at the bottom of the ingredients list to fool the consumer into thinking it is just a small amount?

A: Federal regulations require ingredients to be listed on product labels in descending order by quantity. The ingredient used in the highest amount (such as water) is usually found at the start of the list, while additives and fragrances that are used in small amounts are placed at the end of the list. These ingredient lists apply only to retail products intended for home use. Any other products, including those used by beauticians in salons, those labeled "For Professional Use Only," and cosmetic samples given out by department stores and hotels, don't need to include the ingredient declaration. They must, however, state the distributor, list the content's quantity, and include any warning statements for the customer's protection.

Q: I'm confused. When I try to look up medical information on the Internet, I get so many sites claiming they have the hottest medical breakthrough and the products to go with it. How can I separate truth from fiction?

A: Don't get bamboozled on the Web. Many sites are backed by product manufacturers with only one thing in mind: to get you to buy their

Quick Tip

If you think you've been duped by false advertising, speak out. Complain to your local FDA office or call the FDA's Office of Consumer Affairs at 800-532-4440.

products, whether it's the latest herbal remedy or a "medicine." Also, beware of any "medical breakthrough" testimonials or treatments based only on anecdotal (not peer-reviewed) reports. Therapies that work have been researched and printed in medical journals (or at least on the front page of the *New York Times*).

Q: I've been reading about skin care products with HGH (Human Growth Hormone), DHEA, and pregnenolene. All these products supposedly are hormones that strengthen the skin and make it less prone to wrinkling. Should I go out and get them to look younger?

A: Hold on to your wallet. Cosmetics claims aren't regulated by the FDA, so you should wait until a bit more conclusive research evidence on these products comes to the forefront. (Remember: peer-reviewed studies are a good bet that the products are safe and effective.) In the meanwhile, be careful about playing around with hormones. In fact, large doses of the hormone DHEA may be linked to acne and increased facial hair growth. Stick with the products we know can help safely reduce the effects of aging, such as sunscreens, antioxidants, and vitamin A–derivative products.

chapter nineteen

Hair Repair

*Some people weave burlap into the fabric of our lives,
and some weave gold thread. Both contribute to
make the whole picture beautiful and unique.*

—ANONYMOUS

Healthy Hair

More than many other parts of their body or appearance, it seems, many people
are most conscious about their hair, particularly if they feel they're losing it! A
common reason for a visit to a dermatologist is when people notice that their hair
is thinning or falling out. This sometimes seems to be more troublesome to both
men and women than other signs of aging. When going over hair loss with my
patients, this is what we discuss.

Reasons for Hair Loss

Hair loss can be due to many factors. Postpartum hair loss often occurs in the
first few months after delivery due to falling hormone levels and the stress of
delivery and usually corrects itself as the hormone levels return to normal. People
often see significant hair loss 3 to 6 months after surgery or a traumatic or stressful
event. Of course, hair that is subjected to harsh treatment, like repeated coloring
and/or bleaching in quick succession, is fragile and likely to break, which often is
mistaken for hair that is falling out due to hormonal reasons. I often ask the patient
to have some blood work done; low-functioning thyroids are often responsible for
hair loss, as are changing hormone levels.

After we discuss the possible reasons for the perceived hair loss, I do a simple
test to see if the hair actually *is* falling out. I pull gently on a small section of hair,
and if fewer than five hairs come out in my fingers with each pull, the hair loss is
within the normal range. I usually try to educate patients about what normal hair
loss looks like. It is normal to lose a hundred hairs per day! Now, if you have long

hair, this may look like a lot when you see it on the bathroom floor. If you truly think your hair is falling out, you have to actually collect and count all of the hair that falls out in one 24-hour period–that means collecting the hair out of the drain, off the floor, out of your hairbrush, and off your clothing. Yes, it is annoying but it's the only way to truly count.

What To Do?

If I reach a conclusion that the patient really is experiencing hair loss or thinning, then I see if we can do anything about it. Hair loss due to pregnancy, post-trauma, or harsh treatment will often resolve on its own (with gentle treatment in the meantime). If the blood tests reveal something out of the normal range (such as low iron or thyroid levels), medications, diet supplements, or other testing may be indicated. If the hair loss is genetic, and much of it is, Rogaine (topically applied minoxidil, an over-the-counter preparation) is appropriate for women as well as men. Propecia (an oral medication), while not indicated for use by women by the manufacturer, is in my opinion also safe for women as long as they do not become pregnant while taking it. Daily multivitamins and biotin supplements are also safe and helpful.

Hair Beauty

Ask any woman what one of her most important beauty assets is, and she'll tell you it is her hair. The way you cut, shampoo, color, and blow-dry your hair, as well as its health, affect the way your hair looks. I asked a few experts for advice outside my arena: Sheree Ladove for advice on shampoo ingredients, David Kastin of Arrojo Cutler Salon in New York City for information on how to blow-dry your hair, and Borja of Borja Color Studio in New York City for advice on highlighting and coloring your hair to suit your face.

Ingredients Watch

All shampoos contain surfactants or surface-active agents, which are what actually cleanse the hair. Some surfactants are better than others when it comes to shampoo formulations, suggests Sheree Ladove.

Ingredients to avoid include common chemical preservatives, such as ammonium lauryl sulfate and ammonium laureth sulfate. Low-budget shampoos often contain these harsh ingredients because they are inexpensive and create a very foamy lather.

The very worst ingredient to find its way into a shampoo is sodium C-14-16 olefin sulfonate, a really harsh chemical that strips the hair of color and is found in many cheap shampoos. You also need to watch out for sodium chloride–table salt–in the ingredient list. It's a cheap ingredient to thicken shampoo and strips the hair of oils.

For best benefits, look for botanical-based products with natural surfactants. Here are some natural surfactants to look for in a shampoo:

Avocado
Borage oil
Cocomido propyl betaine (often used in baby shampoo)
Grapeseed oil (an excellent antioxidant that also helps protect hair color)
Kukui nut
Macadamia nut oil (gives hair great shine)
Meadow foam seed oil
Sunflower oil
Wheatgerm oil

Pass the Hair Test

Choose from the following ways to treat your hair's condition:

Oily hair: Hair that appears greasy less than 24 hours after washing is oily. Shampoos for all hair types should be gentle, but with oily hair you need to wash more often and lather twice. It is also possible to have hair that is oily near the scalp but dry near the ends; if so, use conditioner on the ends only. Make sure any styling products you use are oil free.

Dry hair: If your hair looks frizzy and tangles easily, it is probably dry. Use a shampoo designed for dry hair that has a lower concentration of cleansing ingredients and lots of moisturizing ingredients. Drinking enough water, eating a diet that's not ultra-low in fats, and using a humidifier may all help improve dry hair.

Note: Don't confuse dry hair with dry scalp. You may have seborrheic dermatitis (a kind of dandruff) or even psoriasis, both of which can be treated with medicated shampoos and/or other topical medications. In fact, any hair type may have these conditions.

Fine hair: Thin, flyaway hair may benefit from "volumizing" products (shampoos, conditioners, and styling products). They contain an amino acid that helps bulk up the hair shaft. Panthenol, another ingredient, coats the hair shaft to help amplify it. Use a minimum of conditioner and styling products, however; even the most volumizing ingredients can still weigh hair down if used excessively.

Color-treated hair: The staying power of your color processing can be extended by using specially formulated shampoos for color-treated hair. If possible, look for a pH factor of 5.2 to 5.6 to neutralize the alkalinity of hair dye. Keep your hair protected from the sun (with a scarf or hat) to avoid "brassiness" and other color changes.

Myth: You should brush your hair 100 strokes a day to keep it silky and shiny.

FACT: To bring out the shine in your hair, you need to increase blood circulation in the scalp and stimulate scalp oils—by brushing your hair just 15 to 20 strokes a day. If you brush more than that, you risk breaking the hair and possibly even losing more hair than you normally do a day.

Not All for One

You may be tempted to save time and money by using a shampoo/conditioner combo. If so, you may want to rethink your strategy. All-in-one products are very bad for your hair and skin because they use large amounts of silicones (in laminate gels), which coat the hair shaft and smooth it down. While this may seem to "tame" your locks, it doesn't really clean your hair. Women who use these products often run into trouble getting perms to take because the hair is so coated with silcone, the perm just won't work.

The bottom line with a shampoo: Check the ingredients. The first ingredient of a good shampoo should always be water. Contrary to popular belief, your shampoo can also contain alcohol, which is a preservative, but it should rank as the third or fourth–never the first–ingredient. Without exception, water should reign at the top of your shampoo's ingredient list.

Advice on How to Blow-Dry Your Hair

Ever notice how you can never get your hair to look like it does just after you step out of the salon? That's because the pros take a lot of time and use the best tools to get your hair looking its best. Taking a little time to dry your hair correctly instead of running out the door with a wet head can really enhance your hairstyle and appearance. The correct blow-drying method depends, in part, on your hair type and desired style. Follow these styling tips from David Kastin:

Tricks of the Trade

For straight hair styles:

Step 1: Apply a volumizing or hair-styling product to the roots of towel-dried hair. Comb the volumizer through to the ends.

Step 2: Part your hair where you normally do, then separate it into four sections, using clips to keep each section in place. Working in sections, unclip hair and dry the bottom layers first before moving to the top layers.

Step 3: Use a brush to lift up hair and move the brush and hair dryer together along the hair shaft, from the scalp to the ends (where you can curl the ends under if you like). Prevent frizzing by holding the dryer eight inches away and by keeping it pointed down the hair shaft. This keeps the hair's cuticles flat and smooth, enabling your hair to better reflect light. The result: lots of sexy shine.

Step 4: Bend forward and flip hair over, aiming the nozzle at the roots at the nape of the neck–this creates "lift" and movement. Turn off the dryer, flip your hair back as you stand up, and lightly smooth the top layers of the hair, with either your brush or fingers. Spray lightly with hair spray to set the style.

For curly hair:

Note: The above also applies to curly hair that you want to blow straight. Use a straightening or smoothing hair product and a paddle brush to achieve a smooth look.

To keep or enhance a curly style:

Step 1: Use a light mousse or gel so as to not weigh hair down. Use a diffuser on your hair dryer and style with your fingers as opposed to a brush.

Step 2: After hair is dry, apply a shine product to your hands and "scrunch" into the curls to hold the style.

The Right Brush

David Kastin says that using the right brush helps tremendously in achieving beautiful results. He feels that spending a few dollars on quality tools is worth the investment. Here's the rundown:

Vent Brushes: On these brushes, the body of the brush (where the bristles are anchored) is open, allowing air from the dryer to flow through. Great for almost any style. For long hair, simply wrap around the brush to pull out any curl as you dry.

Rolling Brushes: Great for turning ends under (or out, for a flip style). For shorter hair, choose a brush with a smaller diameter, so hair can wrap completely around it.

Paddle Brushes: Great for smoothing out large sections of hair or straightening curly hair. Because the bristles are widely spaced, air flows between them, creating fullness for fine hair.

Natural Bristle Brushes: Can be found on all shapes of brushes. Helps to control static, often caused by plastic and nylon bristles.

Styling Products

Pro Styling Tips

According to David Kastin, another one of your tools is the right styling product. It will help achieve the look you want and hold your style together.

Gel: Thick, usually oil-free styling product to be worked into wet hair before styling. Results in a smooth look when used with a hair dryer or can be left on wet hair for the "wet look." Good for most hair types, gel also comes in a spray form.

Mousse: Lighter formulation, usually dispenses from an aerosol-type container. Good for thin or fine hair due to its light consistency, though it's probably not strong enough to keep curly hair straight.

Quick Tip

Want to hold hair in place without the stiffness of gel or spray? Kastin suggests you mix together a dab of gel with a dab of conditioner (just a fingerful of each) then rub into the palms and run through your hair. The conditioner dilutes the thickness of the gel, while the gel seals in the conditioner's moisturizing ability.

Volumizer: May come in a spray, gel, or mousse form. Coats the hair to create a thicker appearance and "pump up the volume."

Shine products: Add shine and conditioning to dry or dull hair. They can be used before or after styling.

Pomades: Thick creams or gels, sometimes even with a waxy consistency, they hold curls and short styles in place with a very moisturized look. Often used on men's styles.

Frizz tamer's: A newer entry into stylists' toolboxes, used to add humectants to define curls, keep straight styles smooth, and keep the frizzies at bay.

Permanent Changes

Of course, most women are familiar with permanents. Once the domain of little old ladies, perms have evolved with the times and are available both in salons and as at-home formulas. A good perm won't fry your hair but will create permanent curls or waves to create a different look (of course, it's only as permanent as the hair it curls; as the hair grows out, so does the perm). Straightening hair is back in vogue as well, with certain Hollywood stars popularizing the straight-hair look. Both use chemical processes to alter the hair's structure and can be a look unto themselves or can be used to create a particular hairstyle.

The Color Conundrum

According to research conducted by L'Oréal, 56 percent of women over the age of 16 color their hair. That's a lot of you! Color changes are easy and fun and go a long way toward keeping a youthful appearance. Whether you choose to have your hair colored by a professional in a salon or do it yourself at home, here are a few general pointers for best results:

Unless you *want* a very drastic change all at once (and some do), choose a color not too far from your natural color, or color in stages if you want to make a big change. If all you want to do is cover gray, choose a shade close to your natural color and do it before your hair is mostly gray.

As women age, their hair color should lighten accordingly. Older women can look unnatural with jet black hair.

Try to choose a color that matches your skin tone.

Borja's Guide to Choosing a Color

Choosing hair color to complement your skin tone is not hard. First of all, anything goes these days, so whatever *you* really like, even if it doesn't follow "the rules," is fine. In general, however:

Fair skin tones can have blonde, red, brown, or black hair, but it's the undercolor that will complement the skin; stay away from ash undertones and go for warm, golden tones in the blonde, brunette, and red shades.

Olive skin looks best with cool colors in neutral blonde, rich brown, or black shades to minimize the yellow undertone (think Mediterranean).

Dark skin, from Latina to black, should stick to dark shades, either brunette or black, but red undertones and some highlights can look great.

Asian skin looks most natural with dark hair, but undertones of burgundy, blue/black or even a golden brown add excitement and dimension.

Borja says that highlighting your hair adds a whole new range of possibilities, as do lowlights (darkening sections of hair within a color range to add depth). Lightening the hair near the face opens up that area, drawing attention to it; darker colors conceal. Here are some other highlighting guidelines:

Natural blondes look good with golden to pale ivory highlights.
Brunettes can lighten up with deep chestnut to soft amber accents.
Redheads brighten with strawberry blonde to gold tones.
Dark hair looks best with dark red-toned shades, but dramatic blond highlights are in now too.

Highlights can also accentuate a good feature or create an illusion, suggests Borja. Highlights around the eye area and at the temples open up and draw attention to the eyes. To slim a round face, use lowlights, or darker tones, around the face to create slimming shadows. Highlights should be placed mainly at the top of the head and forehead to elongate the face. To camouflage a large nose, part hair on the side and use bold, chunky highlights placed all over to draw attention away from the center of the face. A small face gets height, with highlights on the crown and bang area. Highlights around the sides open up the face further. Long faces are broadened when highlights are added around the temples and sides of the face. The crown area should be left darker.

Borja's Tips on Choosing the Right Coloring Formula

Hair color comes in different formulas that produce different results, mostly in terms of how long they last.

Temporary: These color treatments can come as a rinse, mousse, shampoo-in, or conditioner, and work best when you want a quick, short-lived change. It's also a good way to "try out" a hair color if you're nervous or a first timer. Because they don't penetrate the hair, they rinse away with the next couple of shampoos.

Semi-Permanent: These color treatments change your natural shade without lightening your hair. Since they don't contain peroxide or ammonia, they don't lighten hair but can be used to try a dark color. A semi-permanent color treatment lasts for up to 12 shampoos.

Demi-Permanent: These long-lasting semi-permanent coloring products actually contain a small amount of peroxide, so they slightly lighten hair while also depositing color. This type of product doesn't contain ammonia, however, so it won't lighten hair significantly. When you use it to cover gray, it will look like subtle highlights. Demi-permanent color treatments last through 20 to 30 shampoos.

Permanent: Choose this when you're ready for a long-lasting change. Because this type of coloring treatment contains peroxide and ammonia, it strips color from the hair and then deposits a new shade on the hair shaft. The color lasts until the hair that was colored grows out (which means you need to touch up the roots periodically!).

Home vs. Salon

According to the same L'Oréal study mentioned earlier, 40 percent of the women who do color their hair have done so at home at one time or another. Here are the pros and cons of home versus salon coloring:

Salons:
Pros:
- Custom blending
- More refined colors, shades, and blending of highlights
- Less likelihood of color mishaps, from a bad result to a chemical reaction, in the hands of a professional
- The pampering atmosphere of a salon

Cons:
- More expensive than coloring at home
- More time consuming
- Results, especially with the semi-permanent formulations, are not necessarily better than what you'd get at home
- Stylists may pressure you to do something trendy or that you don't really want to do

Home Coloring:
Pros:
- Less expensive and time consuming
- You don't need an appointment
- You can watch "Friends" in your bathrobe and drink tea while the color sets

Cons:
- More likelihood of adverse chemical reaction, especially if you color on top of a perm or if directions are not followed precisely
- Difficult to combine color treatments with highlights
- Can be messy and smelly

Note: Applying any chemical process to your hair always carries the risk of an adverse reaction, ranging from but not limited to an irritated scalp, chemical burns, and brittle hair. Semi-permanent dye does not affect the structure of the hair, but permanent dye integrates into the hair, weakens the shaft, and can result in fractured or broken hairs. There is also an ingredient in most hair color products that some people are allergic to, called PPPD or para-phenylenediamine. If you are allergic to this ingredient, you are out of luck as far as dark hair colors go but can probably highlight your hair, since that is a process of removing color and not adding color.

After-Color Care by Borja

Don't brush: Since coloring leaves the hair temporarily weakened, use a wide-tooth comb and not a brush to detangle wet hair after shampooing.

Make the switch: Use a shampoo, conditioner, and styling products that are specially formulated for color-treated hair to help extend the life of the color.

Watch out: Chlorine can turn even natural blonde hair a greenish hue and can even straighten permed hair; always rinse your hair in clean water after swimming in a pool.

Beware of the sun: Sun exposure is not only damaging to your skin but to your hair as well. Keep hair covered with a scarf or hat whenever possible to keep it healthy.

chapter twenty

The Power of a Smile

Start off every day with a smile and get it over with.
—ANONYMOUS

GLOWING SKIN CAN MAKE YOU LOOK YEARS YOUNGER. CAN YOU GUESS ANOTHER great way to take years off your face? It's as simple as making cosmetic changes to your teeth. That's right: Laminate veneering, bonding, or whitening teeth can make a huge difference in the way you look and, ultimately, in the way you feel about yourself.

Because a nice smile has served as an invitation to social and professional success from time immemorial, I wanted to give you the most up-to-date information on what you need to do to get yours in prime working order. For that advice, I went to Dr. Linda Golden, a cosmetic dentist based in Manhasset, New York, whom the *New York Times* has featured as an expert in her craft. Here, she reveals the secrets to a better smile—and a younger-looking face.

Men and women constantly strive to improve their looks. We work out to improve our muscle tone. We dress to flatter our shapes. We get the hippest hair cuts and the most becoming hair colors. Makeup artists show us how to chisel our cheekbones and to make the most of our facial features. We gladly submit to chemical peels, microdermabrasion, liposuction, and whatever nips and tucks we deem necessary to achieve our own best image of ourselves.

So why not beautify our smiles? After all, people from the beginning of time have responded to a happy, reassuring smile. Why not let them respond to yours?

Your smile is a gift you give to the people you come into contact with every day. When you meet someone for the first time, your smile instantly communicates your good intentions and lack of hostility. It demonstrates in the most natural way possible that you want your experience with this person to be a pleasant one. If someone is already your friend, your smile communicates warmth, playfulness, good humor, and understanding. To someone you love, a smile can say what words cannot. It says with certainty that you are exactly where and with whom you want to be.

Smile for Your Life

Smiling is good for your health and well-being. In fact, psychologists say that smiling not only reduces stress, it also releases endorphins, which give you a feeling of well-being.

Because smiles make everyone happy all around, if you feel the need to cover up or hide your smile you are robbing yourself of one of the healthiest, most beneficial drawing (or calling) cards available. If you are uncomfortable with the appearance of your smile because your teeth are crooked or broken or discolored, you may subconsciously use gestures to hide them, such as covering your mouth or lips with your hands as you talk, smiling tightly, or doing something to distract the focus from your face (such as gesturing wildly or twirling your hair). These gestures are self-defeating and don't really fool anyone. If you are careful about how and when you show your teeth, your guarded smile may make other people feel you are unfriendly or uptight.

The people you encounter daily respond constantly to the subtle clues you give off. If you talk with your lips pursed, for example, people may feel you are hiding secrets from them. Placing your hand over your mouth when you smile or talk may make people think you lack confidence in other areas of your life. It may even make people feel you are unapproachable or, worse, nervous or angry at them.

It's a fact of life: If you want to look your best, but you feel that your teeth are holding you back, you've got to make a change.

Get a Smile Makeover

If you look back at older photos of celebrities, you'll notice that, as most of them achieve fame, they leave behind their old set of teeth in favor of a brand-new (usually whiter and larger) set of chops with star power. But redesigning teeth isn't just for celebrities.

A good cosmetic dentist can redesign anyone's teeth and provide a list of options to suit any budget. A good cosmetic dentist will work with patients to help them become their best selves and to let their individual personalities shine through their equally individual smiles. The transformation (as you will see) can be dramatic.

Patient Profiles

Here are a number of Dr. Golden's patients and their stories, to show how well cosmetic dentistry works.

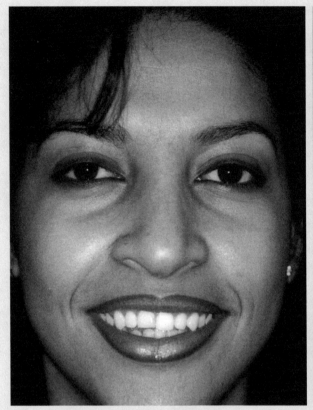 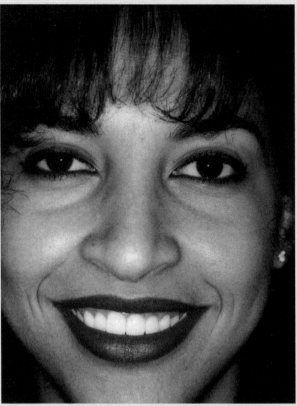

BEFORE: PULY'S TEETH WERE CHIPPED, CROOKED AND YELLOW, WITH AN OPEN BITE.

AFTER: VENEERING ON ALL SIX OF HER FRONT TEETH, HELPED PULY ACHIEVE A BETTER COLOR, AND CLOSED UP HER OPEN BITE.

Puly

BEFORE: This attractive, young hairdresser always smiled at people, but told me she was unhappy with the way her smile looked.

PROBLEM: Puly's teeth were chipped, crooked,and yellow. She also had an open bite on her right side.

SOLUTIONS: Puly chose veneers for all six of her front teeth, for several reasons:

- To achieve a better color
- To close up Puly's bite, so less of her tongue showed
- To protect the teeth that were chipping.

Puly reports that all her clients ask how she got such a beautiful smile.

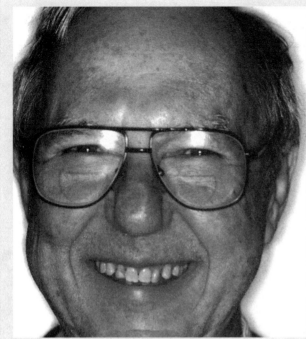

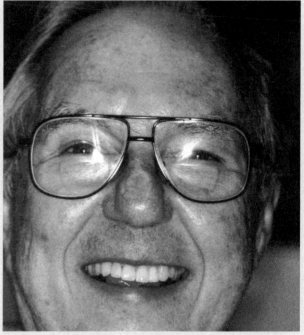

BEFORE: JIM HAS WORN DOWN CHIPPED, CROOKED TEETH BEFORE GETTING OLD FILLINGS REMOVED, AND HAVING SEVEN VENEERS APPLIED.

AFTER: PATIENT AFTER PROCEDURE HAS HIS SMILE RESTORED.

Jim

BEFORE: Jim is an attractive gentleman who had a tremendous amount of staining from smoking and the accumulated effects of aging.

PROBLEMS: Jim had several dental problems:

- Staining
- Chipped teeth
- Crooked teeth
- Old fillings and bondings that needed to be replaced.

SOLUTIONS: Restoring Jim's smile required several steps:

- Removing all of Jim's old restorations, fillings, and bondings.
- Applying veneers to seven teeth.
- Replacing one crown (the replaced crown was unstable, due to the lack of remaining tooth structure)
- Choosing a natural color for the veneers and the crown to match his other teeth (which meant allowing for some staining), because Jim didn't choose to correct his lower teeth at the time.

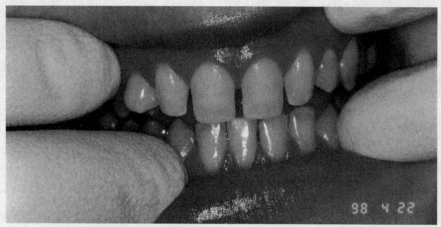

BEFORE: DIANE HAS DISCOLORED, UNEVENLY SPACED, MISSHAPEN TEETH BEFORE GETTING VENEERS TO CORRECT THE COLOR, SHAPE OF TEETH, AND IRREGULAR SPACING.

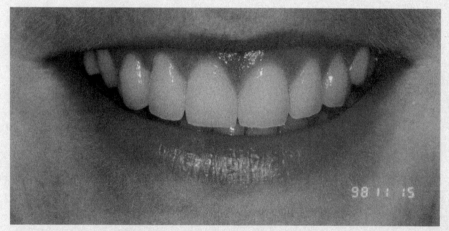

AFTER: THIS BRIDE-TO-BE GETS A BETTER SMILE FOR HER WEDDING PRESENT AFTER GETTING VENEERS.

Diane

BEFORE: This bride-to-be wanted a better smile for her wedding.

PROBLEM: Diane had discoloration, spacing problems, and misshapen teeth.

SOLUTION: Veneers were placed to correct the color, shape, and irregular spacing of her teeth.

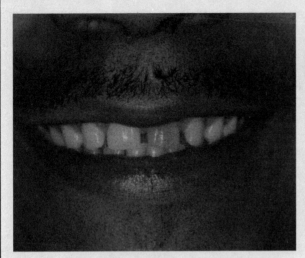

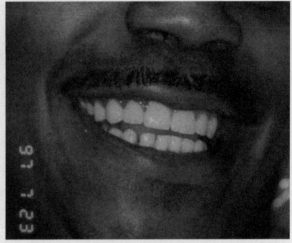

BEFORE: TRACY HAD A SEVERELY DISCOLORED FRONT TOOTH AND SIGNIFICANT SPACING.

AFTER: PATIENT AFTER HAVING HIS FRONT TOOTH BLEACHED, AND AFTER VENEERS WERE PLACED ON THE TOP EIGHT TEETH, CLOSING THE SPACES, BUT LEAVING A SLIGHT SPACE BETWEEN THE TWO FRONT TEETH FOR A NATURAL LOOK.

Tracy

BEFORE: Tracy was concerned about his appearance, because he was picked up for a second season on *Saturday Night Live,* and wanted to look good, but not change his look too much so people would still recognize him.

PROBLEM: He had a discolored front tooth and his teeth were unevenly spaced.

SOLUTION:
- Tracy's discolored front tooth was internally bleached.
- His other teeth were bleached using a home bleaching method.
- Veneers were placed on his top eight teeth.
- The veneers helped close the spacing between his teeth.
- A slight space was left between his two front teeth to keep his look natural–and recognizable.

Top Treatments for Restoring and Redesigning Your Smile

Today, you can choose from several cosmetic dental procedures to ensure a better, prettier smile. Let's go over the most common ones, in order of complexity (from least to most complex).

Tooth Whitening Guide

As you age, your teeth tend to yellow and discolor slightly. (Drinking coffee and tea and eating foods like berries certainly doesn't help.) You can try a whitening toothpaste, but if it doesn't do the trick, check out what a cosmetic dentist can do for you. One popular method that could boost your smile's dazzle is bleaching. This technique works best on nicely shaped teeth that are not marred by extensive yellow/orange or gray discoloring. In some cases, but not all, teeth that have been stained by tetracycline can also be bleached. Still, most teeth are bleachable to some degree. Three bleaching methods are currently available.

Laser Bleaching

Where It's Done: In the dentist's office. Specific dental offices have a laser for whitening.

What It Is: First, teeth are isolated for treatment, with a dental dam, to minimize leakage of oxidizing agents into other areas of the mouth. The teeth are then prepared by "painting" them with a special acid, which is combined with a concentrated hydrogen peroxide solution (as high as 50 percent). Your dentist then uses a laser beam to painlessly activate the bleach. At-home maintenance treatments are often used to prolong the effects of laser bleaching.

Strengths:

- This is the quickest method of brightening and whitening teeth.
- No at-home trays (although some offices include an at-home kit for touch-ups).

The combination of the pretreatment and laser creates a reaction that eliminates the staining in the pores of the teeth. For the laser bleaching, a chemical oxidizing agent–normally hydrogen peroxide or carbamide per-oxide–is introduced into the pores of the teeth to eliminate the stain. Toothpaste uses a much weaker strength and there is no reactive agent in the toothpaste.

When Do You See Results: Immediately

Did you know that...

In the 1700s, toothbrushes were made from the hair of hogs, badgers, and horses.

Weaknesses:

* Relapse; as teeth become stained again over time, rebleaching is required.
* Increased sensitivity (in some patients).
* Results may vary.
* Patients with exposed root structure or generally sensitive teeth usually experience heightened sensitivity during the procedure.
* Fillings, crowns, and veneers will not lighten, so they usually need to be replaced to match the rest of the mouth.
* Some darkening may appear in about a year.

Cost: $1,200 to $1,500

Power Bleaching
Where It's Done: In the dentist's office
What It Is: A process similar to laser bleaching, power bleaching uses an acid and hydrogen peroxide solution that is activated by a high-intensity light (rather than by a laser).
Strengths:
* Like laser bleaching, this process works quickly to eliminate staining from the pores of teeth.
* Power bleaching uses high-strength solutions—as much as 50 percent hydrogen peroxide to 44 percent carbamide peroxide.
* Fast results. No at-home trays.
When Do You See Results: Immediately.
Weaknesses:

* May require several visits and long sessions.
* Increased sensitivity.
* Must do home bleaching to maintain the effects.
* Results vary.

Cost: $250 to $400 per treatment; usually requires several treatments. Also requires additional cost of at-home treatments to maintain effects.

Home Bleaching
Where It's Done: First in the dentist's office, then primarily at home, with observation visits to the dentist.
What It Is: With at-home bleaching, the dentist makes a plaster mold in the exact shape of the patient's teeth. From this mold, a plastic tray is fabricated that fits over the teeth; a compartment inside the tray holds a solution of carbamide peroxide (in a 10 percent to 22 percent solution). The patient wears this tray, filled with solution, for approximately four to six hours (during the day or while sleeping), depending on the brand of bleaching for-

mula used. (Treatment time varies according to the manufacturer.) A variety of treatment options accommodate different patients' needs, for example, allowing for day bleaching twice a day for 30 minutes or for bleaching while you sleep. Either of the two other bleaching techniques can be combined with home bleaching.

Strengths:

- The latest research suggests that at-home bleaching is perhaps the safest and most effective of the bleaching methods.
- No rubber dams.
- Minimal chair time.
- Trays can be used over a long span of time.
- Fewer office visits are required.
- Less sensitivity.
- Home bleaching is generally the most affordable method of bleaching. The bulk of the initial cost is for the mold, which can be used repeatedly for touch-ups over several years. The cost of refill solution is relatively nominal.

When Do You See Results: One week to 10 days, sometimes sooner. Results vary greatly, depending on the type of stains and or patient's compliance with the dentist's instruction. Yellow and brown stains bleach best. Grays are more difficult, and tetracycline staining can be reduced over a few months.

Weaknesses:

- Requires periodic touch-ups.
- For best results, the bleaching technique must be repeated once every six months to two years.
- If the patient is a smoker or has a penchant for coffee or red wine, the process most likely will need to be repeated more frequently.
- Patients need to be compliant—noncompliance can lead to disappointing results.
- Less rapid results.
- Length of time required is usually two weeks or more.
- You have to wear something on your teeth for hours a day or at night.
- Patients do not like the taste.
- Results vary.

Cost: $500 to $800 a kit; $20 to $30 for each gel refill (touch-ups)

Bonding

Where It's Done: In the dentist's office.

What It Is: Bonding involves adhering a layer of plastic, called a composite, to the teeth to make them more attractive. It is a good choice for patients who want to change the shape, structure, and/or surface of their teeth. First, the dentist performs some minimal drilling directly on the enamel of the tooth to prepare it for the bonding composite material. Next, a mild acid is used to condition the surface of the teeth (which is necessary to adhere the bonding to the enamel), and the composite is placed on the tooth. Then, a high-intensity light is directed on the teeth to harden the material. Finally, the dentist contours, sculpts, and polishes the material to create the desired shape and length.

Strengths:

- Bonding is a wonderful technique for repairing chipped or fractured teeth.
- Bonding can also do great things for pitted or spotted teeth.
- Bonding can be used to close unwanted spaces between the teeth or to give crooked teeth the illusion of being straighter.
- In more extreme cases, bonding can completely cover the surface of each tooth to mask discoloration, bad positioning, or poor shape.
- A patient's teeth can also be lightened during the same office visit.
- The procedure is usually painless, and consequently most treatments require no anesthesia (depending, of course, on the patient's tolerance).
- One advantage of bonding is that this procedure usually requires minimal tooth reduction (read, drilling).
- Bonding is one of the more affordable of the cosmetic procedures.

When Do You See Results: Immediately.
Weaknesses:

- The primary downside of bonding is that it is not permanent. The typical bond lasts three to five years.
- You don't get as good a shine and translucency as you do with porcelain laminates.
- Tends to chip easily.
- Stains require routine maintenance.
- It is difficult to acquire a translucency and luster that properly approximate natural teeth, which limits the aesthetic use of bonding.

Cost: $300 to $400 per tooth

Laminate Veneers

Where It's Done: In the dentist's office.
What It Is: If cost is less of a concern and optimal aesthetics are of paramount importance, the top treatment option is most certainly laminate veneers. Laminate veneers are the Rolls-Royce of dentistry: ultra-thin sculpted pieces of tooth-shaped porcelain that fit over the front of your teeth. Veneers

are sort of like jewelry for your teeth—perfect, if your teeth are significantly discolored, chipped, pitted, malformed, or crooked, or if you have unwanted spaces.

This two-step process requires anesthesia and is usually performed on two separate days: On the first visit, the teeth are prepared; on the second visit, the laminates are applied. The process works as follows:

- In preparing the tooth for the procedure, the dentist frequently removes certain parts of the tooth's structure to ensure the sculpted piece of porcelain will fit properly. An impression is taken and the porcelain is sculpted directly on the individual's teeth like a piece of jewelry.
- The teeth receiving the porcelain veneers are chemically treated with the same mild acid used in bonding.
- The tooth-shaped porcelain is then placed on the front of the tooth's surface.
- A high-intensity light is used to adhere the porcelain to the tooth (as with bonding).

Strengths:

- Provides an effective way to change the color, shape, and structure of teeth.
- Good for treating cracks and chips, unwanted gaps between teeth, and crooked teeth.
- Provides a protective covering, where needed, for teeth that have been chipping or wearing away.
- Offers the best option for reshaping or broadening a smile and for creating a younger appearance, because of the life-like luster of the porcelain veneers, which bonding can never achieve.
- Stronger and more permanent than bonding, lasting 10 to 15 years.
- Considerably more stain-resistant than bonding treatments.

When Do You See Results: Immediately after the final (second) treatment, when the veneers are applied.

Weakness: Sometimes previous dental treatment makes it impossible to use laminate veneers. If that is the case, a dentist can redo crown and bridge-work using all porcelain to make it look like the rest of your teeth, matching shape and color.

Cost: Not cheap. $1,000 to $1,500 (or more) per tooth. But they'll last from 10 to 15 years and won't stain.

Porcelain Inlays and Onlays

Where It's Done: In the dentist's office.

What It Is: Old and worn fillings and restorations, such as silver amalgam fillings, which can give teeth a blue tint on the sides, are replaced with porce-

---

Did you know that...

During the sixteenth century, people made their own tooth abrasives, mixing combinations of honey, sugar, crushed bone, and fruit peel.

lain inlays or onlays that closely match the color of your teeth. Porcelain inlays or onlays require isolating teeth, and then drilling out the old fillings under anesthesia. Then an impression is made–like a piece of jewelry in a ceramic studio. On a second visit to the dentist, your teeth are again isolated, you are numbed, and the porcelain is bonded in place, adjusted, and polished. The porcelain onlays are a more conservative procedure than crowning a tooth and can look wonderful used in conjunction with laminate veneers.

Strengths:

- Eliminates the blueish tint from the old silver amalgam fillings.
- Hold up well over time because the adhesion for the bonding provides a strong and strengthening foundation for the teeth.
- Can make a great match to the rest of the teeth.

When Do You See Results: Immediately after the second visit, when the inlays/onlays are applied.

Weaknesses:

- This is an extensive procedure that requires a lot of time. In removing an old restoration, there is always a chance a patient may need a root canal or crown.

Cost: $800 to $1,500 per tooth

How to Create a Younger-Looking Face

When it comes to creating a youthful smile–and face–just remember this: the lips are the curtains, the gums are the scenery, the two front teeth are the stars, and the surrounding teeth are the supporting actors. So:

- The front teeth should be slightly longer than the teeth next to them.
- The smile should broaden as it sweeps toward the back of the mouth. (When you smile, teeth should follow your lip line.)
- There should be no black space in your mouth, in front or in back.
- Teeth should be bright.
- Fix chips and cracks.

Your teeth can also be customized to fit your face shape. For example:

Round Face: Teeth should be slightly square to create a more angular look.
Square Face: Teeth should be more oval-shaped to soften the face.
Heart Face: The central incisors should be flatter across.
Long Face: The smile should be as wide as possible.

chapter twenty-one

Makeup Magic

> *Though we travel the world over to find the beautiful,*
> *we must carry it with us or we find it not.*
>
> —Ralph Waldo Emerson

Using a combination of bleaching, porcelain veneers, and porcelain onlays/inlays, you can get outstanding results and a dazzling smile. Aren't you worth it?

When it comes to advice on new makeup styles and techniques, makeup artist Kimara Ahnert has established a reputation as one of New York City's most prominent makeup artists. Since opening the Kimara Ahnert studio in December 1997, Kimara Ahnert has been hailed as the "Best Makeover in New York" by *New York* magazine and featured in *Vogue, Town & Country, Self,* and *Elle.*

Kimara's Makeup Advice

- Give your skin the subtle sheen of a Hollywood star with Circle of Beauty's Skin Image Highlighter, which creates a beautiful glaze over bare skin or foundation. Another one to try: Lightning by Benefit or Face and Body Powder by L'Oréal. Use shimmer or glow products to accent tops of cheekbones and outer corner of the eyes, and on the shoulders.
- Open up eyes with a white or silver dot of shadow or shimmer in the inner corners.
- Make your own bronzing powder by taking regular body lotion and mixing in a shimmery powder. For fair skin, go to a makeup line that can custom blend a bronzing powder for you, such as Prescriptives. Also, try Physicians Formula Powder Palette Color Corrective Bronzers, which also

come with a color-corrective powder in either green, to neutralize red tones, or mauve, to liven up yellow-toned skin.

- Use a color-correcting concealer under the eyes to neutralize the area. To make eyes pop, use concealer on top before you apply shadow. Some of the newer cream-based shades work better than powder shadows because they provide the illusion of a smoother lid.
- Try shadow instead of eyeliner to line eyes. Shadow is great to use as liner because it is water-resistant. Wet the tip of the brush and use it to line around the eyes as well as on top of the lid, right above eyelashes, for smoky appeal.
- For bigger eyes, draw a line directly under the brow with a fat concealer pencil, then blend in with a cotton swab using an up-and-out motion. This acts as a frame to define your brows.
- Brush a tinted brow gel through lashes for a more natural look than mascara. You can also keep brows in place with a bit of hair mousse. Avoid using hair spray on brows; it can clog pores, causing breakouts.
- To create dramatic eyes, glue a few individual lashes (short looks are more natural) on just the outer corners of the eyes.
- To make lips glisten, apply your regular lipstick as you normally do, and then using fingertips dab on a white iridescent eyeshadow over lips to make them look pouty.

Camouflage Your Cosmetic Surgery

Whether you've had laser resurfacing, a face-lift, a nose or eye job, or a peel, you can hide bruises, flaky spots, and discolored skin with makeup. Check out these skin perfecting tips. Note: Clear the use of any postprocedure products with the physician who performs the procedure.

Flaky, Dry, Sensitive Skin: To take care of your skin, wash your face with a gentle cleanser, such as Cetaphil, and lock in moisture with an extra-creamy moisturizer with antioxidants, such as Neutrogena. Make sure to use hypoallergenic products that contain PABA-free sunscreen.

Puffy Eyes: Keep eye gel in the refrigerator for the most cooling treatment. You can leave an eye mask in there as well. Play down puffiness by using soft, matte shadows in neutral shades (peach, taupe, brown) instead of shadows with frost or glimmer, which emphasize puffiness. Line eyes and wear mascara on upper lashes only.

Dark Circles: You need a good creamy concealer with lots of coverage and opacity. If you have circles that are hard to cover or bruising from cosmetic procedures, you first need to neutralize the area and brighten up the blue cast to the skin with a color like mauve. Put the neutralizing color on first—it will cancel out and lighten up the area—then you can put concealer right on top. Blend with your finger or the corner of a clean, dry sponge. Set by dusting a little loose powder all over.

Redness/Laser Results: Dab moisturizer around the area and then paint on a green color concealer (the green neutralizes the redness), such as Physicians Formula Concealer Stick in green. Over that, use a sponge to apply a foundation in your skin tone. Finally, cover with fine powder (try Cornsilk), using a cotton ball.

Scars: Dealing with scars really takes trial and error. Some scars are coverable, and some are better left alone with just a liquid foundation over them. If you are using a foundation stick or camouflage cream, choose a color that matches your skin tone—anything lighter will highlight the imperfection. If the scar is blue/purple, use a mauve color concealer to prime the area and then follow with concealer or foundation.

Bags Under Eyes: Apply a thin coat of foundation with a damp cosmetic sponge. Use a brush to dab concealer in a shade slightly lighter than the foundation at the base of the "bag" where the darkness is most pronounced. Gently blend well.

Freckles/Blotches: Use a matte oil-free foundation for more opaque coverage. Paint a concealer or foundation on top of areas that need additional covering. Set with a powder foundation.

General Coverage: After surgery or any skin care procedure, your regular foundation won't cut it anymore; you need heavier coverage. If you use a foundation and/or concealer, go for one that contains SPF and is heavy, like Dermablend. For best results, paint it on with a brush and pat it on with your finger or a sponge.

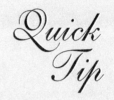

Quick Tip

If your lips have a blue tint to them, your lipstick may appear darker than it is. To compensate: Kimara suggests you go for slightly lighter tones or blend foundation over lips to prime and lighten lip color.

Kimara's Skin Color Tips

Black Skin
Best Foundation: One with deep yellow tones. Many women with black skin need to use two foundations: one for overall coverage; the other two shades darker than skin tone to balance unevenness around the hairline and the jaw.

Avoid: Colors that are too red.

Best Powder: Translucent, light-bronze loose powder.

Makeup Tip: Use beiges and deep metallic browns, such as copper, bronze, and mahogany, with shimmer in them to open up eyes. Try lipsticks in mocha, beige, coffee, and burgundy shades.

Asian Skin
Best Foundation: Ones that have a little yellow in them to complement the yellow undertones in Asian skin.

Avoid: Pink and orange colors; they can be too harsh.

Best Powder: Translucent loose powder with yellow undertones.

Makeup Tip: Use black or charcoal eyeliner along the upper lid, and silver and iridescent shadows to bring out small, deep-set eyes. Lips look lush in mauve or brown shades.

Foundation Facts by Kimara

There is a foundation to suit every skin type:

Normal/Oily Skin: Use a matte, oil-free liquid to powder foundation, such as Cover Girl Simply Powder Foundation.

Dry/Mature Skin: Use a liquid oil-based foundation or one with light-reflecting particles. Try Max Factor Whipped Creme Makeup or Revlon Age Defying Makeup and Concealer.

Combination Skin: You can use either a matte or a liquid foundation. But you must use some kind of powder to set your makeup on the oilier T-zone of the face.

Kimara's Concealer Power

See what form of concealer meets your needs:

Wands: Offer light coverage (best for evening-out discoloration).

Pots: Usually very opaque (best maximum coverage for problem areas, such as dark, under-eye circles).

Pencils: Can hide well-defined spots and small scars.

Sticks: Best when used all over the face.

Tubes: The thick consistency makes these concealers perfect for covering blemishes.

Kimara's Eye Openers

Follow this advice no matter what shape your eyes are.

Small Eyes

To make them bigger, use a lighter color on the lid, and contour in the crease with a medium shade. Wear your eyeliner on either the top or bottom lid, but not on both. Curl lashes with an eyelash curler and then sweep mascara on top lashes only.

Close-Together Eyes

Apply shadow on the outer corner of the crease only. Line only the outer half of the eye and sweep mascara on top lashes only. For evening, add a few individual lashes to the outer half of the eye for sexy appeal.

Wide Eyes

If you have a lot of lid space showing, use a medium shade all over the lid. Line the whole eye and apply more mascara to the lashes above the widest part of the eye. Your contour color should start directly where the brow begins, from the inner corner out. Use mascara all over top and bottom lashes.

Almond-Shaped Eyes

This is the perfect eye shape (sort of like having an oval face). With this shape, you can do whatever you want.

Round Eyes

With round-shaped eyes, you want to extend the line. Basically, follow the rules for close-set eyes to bring the look up and out.

Safety Checkup from Kimara

- Discard all eye makeup every six months, especially liquid products. If you get an infection, throw everything out that you use on your eyes and start all over.
- Face Powder and Blush: Replace them every year and whenever you see any flaking or clumping.
- Liquid and Cream Foundations: Replace them every six months, and get rid of them anytime you notice a smell or an oil separation.
- Eye Shadow: Replace them every year.
- Liquid Mascara and Eye Pencils: Get rid of them every three months.
- Lipstick: Pitch them after two years or if the oil beads, the color changes, or it smells bad.
- Nail Polish: Toss if it starts to separate (the oil separates from the rest of the polish).
- Sharing Makeup: Don't do it, ever! Sharing makeup is a surefire way to transfer bacteria.
- Astringents: Don't store astringents near heat; they'll evaporate. Heat can also turn products bad by breaking down the particles. Instead, keep all cosmetics tightly capped or closed, don't add any water, and keep them in a cool place, away from the light.

Did you know that...

Archaeologists have unearthed palettes for grinding and mixing face powder and eye shadow dating back to 6000 B.C.

Quick Tip

At beauty counters, test foundation on your neck rather than on the back of your hand, which can be three shades lighter than your face and neck.

Shop Savvy

- Check out your local cosmetic discounters for deals and steals. Look for holiday-time packages that include everything you need: shadow, blush, liner, lipstick, mascara, and even gloss.
- Get sable or pony brushes for blush, shadow, and powder.
- Use synthetic brushes, which are stiffer, for painting on creams, concealers, and lipsticks.

Kimara Answers Common Questions

Q: My foundation creases and cakes in cold weather. Any suggestions?

A: When the temperature drops, pigments collect in dry, flaky patches, instead of blending into your skin, and can look horrible. The solution: Wear moisturizer underneath your foundation so it goes on smoother. Skip foundation on dry patches around the nose and eyes. Just blend in the foundation from the surrounding area with your fingertip.

Q: What's the best way to cover a zit?

A: Using a brush, dab concealer on the zit only. Don't pat down the cover-up with your finger, or you'll pull it off. Brush on a little loose powder to lightly blend it in.

Q: Can lipstick chap your lips?

A: Yes. Matte lipsticks, which lack certain moisturizing ingredients, tend to leave lips parched, especially in cold weather. Frosted lipsticks and glosses can also be drying to lips. A better choice: lip gloss or a cream-based lipstick fortified with aloe, mineral oil, or vitamin E. To keep lips smooth and supple, always wear lip balm, either on its own or under your lip color. Look for a balm loaded with emollients, such as petrolatum, lanolin, cocoa butter, and shea butter. Try Bare Escentuals Buzz Latte for Lips, which even tastes good. Balms work in two ways: They create a barrier against the harsh elements, and they also seal in the moisture. Don't forget to exfoliate your lips; they've been sapped of moisture through the winter. Use a smear of petroleum jelly or vitamin E oil and a toothbrush.

Q: Is powder the best way to cover up wrinkles and skin imperfections?

A: No. Actually, powder cakes in wrinkles and lines. Powder also soaks up oil and water, two essential moisturizing ingredients for skin. Use oil-based cream foundations on dry or wrinkled skin. Rule of thumb: cover imperfections by using foundation and concealer and apply powder only as a finishing touch. Instead of pressing powder into skin with a powder puff, buff a light-reflecting powder over makeup with a powder brush. (Light-reflecting powders play an optical trick, making wrinkles look less noticeable.)

Q: Do you have any makeup tips for mature skin?

A: Stay away from matte, oil-free foundations. Instead, use something that is water-based, with only a little oil. If you want something moisturizing but not very opaque, try a moisture tint (moisturizer and foundation in one) from Bobbi Brown, Clinique, Laura Mercier, or Chanel. To hide crow's-feet and wrinkles, use an eyeliner brush to paint a light-reflecting concealer or foundation, such as Revlon's Age Defying Makeup, onto lines. Light-reflecting products are formulated with tiny particles that diffuse light, making lines less noticeable.

Q: How can I fix my lip shape?

A: Follow these tips to improve your natural lip line:

- Thin Lips: To make them fuller, draw a line with liner just outside their natural edge, fill in with lip color, and top with gloss.
- Uneven Lips: Line just outside the thinner half and along the edge of the fuller half. Line lower lip as usual and fill in with lipstick.
- Full Lips: If you want to slim them down, use a light layer of foundation to blur the edges. Then, outline lips just inside their natural line and fill in with a dark, matte color (shine just makes lips seem fuller).

Makeup Tips from a Model

Jane Powers-Clothier, a model for more than 12 years with IMG Models, offers some tricks of the trade:

- The best eyelash curler is from Shu Uemura; it has the correct curve. The best way to use it is to curl lashes, apply mascara, let the mascara dry, and then curl again.

Myth:

Preparation H works to shrink wrinkles.

FACT:

Although some models swear by Preparation H as a cure-all ointment for eye bags, wrinkles, and, believe it or not, cellulite, it is just not so. Preparation H is simply an anti-inflammatory product used to shrink hemorrhoidal tissue. Any claim that it can shrink puffiness in or under the skin, which is caused by fat and sagging, is not medically based. The only puffiness that Preparation H might help temporarily shrink in some people is that caused by temporary factors, such as a late night of partying or a meal high in salt (which increases water retention). The typical puffiness caused by fat pads, such as under-eye pouches, can be permanently improved only by surgery (blepharoplasty).

- My favorite mascara is Christian Dior mascara with cashmere: It has a thick, plush wand.
- A well-shaped brow helps define the eyes. Some of my favorite brow pencils include the Shiseido soft brown brow pencil, the François Nars brow pencil with a brush, the Shu Uemura brow liner, and the Chanel sculpting brow pencil with a brush. I also sometimes use MAC eye shadow in a brown shade called Coquette, which I brush over my brows with a stiff, angled brush.
- If you've overplucked your eyebrows and they're growing in kind of straggly, smooth on Vaseline or Elizabeth Arden's 8-hour cream in the direction the brows grow at night.
- I use Stila Lip Rouge pencil, which goes on smoothly like a magic marker. My upper lip is slightly uneven, so I line the top lip a little above the lip line to even it out.
- To make eyes really pop, smooth along the top lash line with a dark neutral powder, such as Coquette from MAC, blending from the lashes up with a short, blunt brush.
- Focus on one area of the face and don't introduce too many colors. If you use dramatic lipstick, keep the eyes neutral (no red lipstick with blue eyeshadow).
- In general, less *is* more–and blend, blend, blend, preferably with your fingertips.

chapter twenty-two

The Future of Beauty

Beauty is nothing other than the promise of happiness.
—STENDHAL

WHAT IS THE FUTURE OF BEAUTY? WHAT ADVANCES IN MEDICINE, TECHNOLOGY, and social and cultural evolution will affect how we look and feel, both in our youth and as we age? Here's what I see as some major trends:

One-Stop Shopping

The wave of the future has already begun. Anything that saves time and is more efficient, in any kind of industry, appeals to customers. This is evident in businesses of all kinds across the nation and around the world.

When I founded what is now The Center for Dermatology, Cosmetic and Laser Surgery, my practice in Mount Kisco, the idea was to offer my patients whatever they need and want in the way of dermatological and cosmetic procedures and treatments. Under one roof, we offer complete dermatological care, plastic surgery, aesthetic treatments, products, and more. You can get a Botox treatment while a doctor checks out that mole on your son's arm you've always been concerned about, then schedule your husband's liposuction consultation and pick up some sunscreen—all in one visit. The concept of offering the best of each specialty with a team approach, for total patient care, is a trend that no business can ignore.

Young Forever

More and more people are having procedures and treatments done at an earlier age. As these procedures become less invasive and time consuming than in past years, and as we as a society are more conscious about our health and appearance, the acceptance and popularity of "getting something done" is growing. The easier

245

and quicker "lunch-time" procedures, such as Botox, microdermabrasion, and collagen fit well into today's busy lifestyles.

Attitudes are also changing about aging. The natural changes in our appearance used to be thought of as part of "aging gracefully." People now challenge that thinking and are working hard to keep their skin and body fit and healthy by whatever means are available. "Letting oneself go" in middle age or later simply isn't an option, but giving mother nature a helping hand is. Taking advantage of the procedures and technology available, both men and women are having preventative procedures done, such as peels to remove accumulated sun damage, and applying topical products to keep skin looking youthful as they age. The acceptance of cosmetic surgery procedures is rising and the quest for beauty and wellness is no longer limited to the dating and mating years.

Cosmetic surgery procedures, once the domain of "ladies of a certain age," are more popular than ever. Liposuction and breast augmentation are two of the fastest-growing cosmetic surgery procedures, crossing all demographic categories. Patients are no longer waiting until their fifties or later to have a face-lift or a blepharoplasty but are extending their youthful looks by doing these procedures in their thirties. Being aware of the dangers of the sun and tanning is another health-conscious change from the "you-look-healthy-with-a-tan" attitude of the past.

Genie in a Bottle

Topical creams that contain vitamins and other natural and synthetic ingredients will offer improved performance and results. The emergence and continued development of "cosmeceuticals," a combination of pharmaceuticals and regular cosmetics, is well established. New oral vitamin supplements will also soon be available to improve our health and appearance, and doctors will be able to individualize a nutrition program to fit each person's needs.

A Shot in Time

There is exciting news regarding growth hormone and its application to health and rejuvenation of the body. Studies are now being done researching the effect of this hormone on normally aging bodies and the possible antiaging benefits. Preliminary reports indicate that it may increase the muscle mass and youthful capabilities that normally diminish as we advance in years. Other hormones are also being studied as to their possible role in the rejuvenation process.

Based on all the exciting developments taking place, there is no reason that you cannot be the person you want to be, in body, mind, and spirit, as well as in the way you choose to look. You can feel healthy and full of vitality with the proper care and intervention and have a youthful appearance to match. Finally, you can have the quality of life you deserve. These are very exciting times, with lots of great advances to look forward to. Enjoy!

afterword

Why Put Off 'Til Tomorrow Looking Better Today?

It's never too late to be what you might have been.
–George Eliot

You've probably finished the book by now (or you're skipping ahead to see how it all turns out). We've covered a lot of ground together in these pages. I've given you a program for your skin type (whether it's oily, acne-prone, combination, normal, dry, sensitive, or sun-damaged). I've given you guidance on your hormonal changes as well as many common skin problems. I've shared with you the ingredients to avoid–and the ones to look for–in the most common–and not so common–skin-care products. I've shown you how to fix your under-eye bags, your sagging skin, and your sallow complexion. I've informed you about the latest cutting-edge medical techniques to reduce signs of aging, and I've even offered you some advice on selecting high-quality, inexpensive products from your local pharmacy. Now, here's my final piece of advice: It's all up to you.

We're Products of Our Culture

If you need any more reason to change, here's a simple fact: Our culture worships at the throne of youth and beauty. And though you may shake your fist at the injustice of it all, it is true. As women and men age, they are forced to compare themselves with the images of youth and beauty repeated in the media–in print, on television, and at the movies. Whether you like it or not, Hollywood keeps raising the bar on beauty. They can, mainly because they have access to the age-proofing techniques and technologies featured in this book. Today, because of laser technology, advances in cosmetic surgery, and the most technological skin-care techniques, a 50-year-old can look 20 years younger, and a 30-year-old can look like she's in her twenties.

Studies throughout the years have shown that attractive women (and tall, attractive men) have been rated as more intelligent and more capable than those who were not up to the traditional standards of beauty. Whatever your age, making sure you look your best gives you all the ammunition you need to fight ageism before it starts—on your own terms.

You can look better—now (with or without surgery)—or you can stay just as you are. If you picked up this book in the first place, it's probably because you had hoped that I would give you a way to turn back the hands of time (or keep them from turning quite as fast as they seem to these days). I've done my part; now it's time for you to do yours. Remember, information is power, and I'm putting this power right into your hands.

Don't you owe it to yourself to give yourself a competitive advantage in the social and professional arena? Don't you owe it to yourself to be the best you can be? Don't you owe it to yourself to have Beautiful Skin?

I think you do. No—I **know** you do.

A final thought:

To laugh often and much; to win the respect of intelligent people and the affection of children; to earn the appreciation of honest critics and endure the betrayal of false friends; to appreciate beauty; to find the best in others; to leave the world a little better, whether by a healthy child, a garden patch or a redeemed social condition; to know even one life has breathed easier because you have lived. This is the meaning of success.

—RALPH WALDO EMERSON

Glossary

The expert at anything was once a beginner.
–HELEN HAYES

Acid: In skin-care terms, anything with a pH 1 to a pH 7. An acid is actually less irritating to skin than an alkalai, because normal skin already has an acidity level (or pH) between 5.5 and 6.5.

Alcohol: Generally, this is a solvent that dissolves oil. However, some alcohol found in skin-care products may actually moisturize, as in the case of cetearyl alcohol and lanolin alcohol. Ethyl alcohol does not moisturize and in high concentrations will dry out the skin.

Alkaline: It is the opposite of acidic and occurs when the pH is greater than 7. The higher the number, the more alkaline the substance. Soaps are alkaline (typically pH 10 to pH 11), which enables soap to remove the dirt trapped in skin, but it can also sometimes irritate skin.

Alpha Hydroxy Acids (AHAs): Naturally occurring compounds found in fruits, wine, sour milk, and sugar cane that help turn over, or exfoliate, the top layer of skin cells, renewing the skin and leaving the complexion smoother and clearer.

Amino Acids: In various combinations, these acids, which are essential for life, form proteins.

Antioxidants: Added to products, foods, and cosmetics to stop deterioration when they are exposed to air. Some antioxidants, such as vitamins A, C, and E, slow down free radicals, which are produced by pollution, the sun, and the environment. If not stopped by antioxidants, these free radicals cause aging, by causing damage to the skin.

Ascorbic Acid: Vitamin C, added to skin-care products as an antioxidant.

Benzoyl Peroxide: This anti-acne drug dries up blemishes and helps eliminate the bacteria that cause pimples. Although it is highly effective, in too strong a concentration (more than 5 percent) it can irritate skin.

Bisabolol: The active ingredient in chamomile flowers, it is soothing to skin.

Ceramides: A structural lipid present in the outer layer of the epidermis (or stratum corneum) that helps retain water in the skin.

Collagen: The protein found in skin and cartilage, which, along with elastin, maintains the skin's elasticity, firmness, and strength.

Comedogenic: A pore-blocking ingredient that can cause breakouts. Products labeled "noncomedogenic" have been tested to show that their ingredients do not block pores.

Dermatologist Tested: Clinically tested with dermatological supervision.

Detergents: These synthesized chemicals lift oils, fat, grime, and other dirt from the skin and hold them in a foam that is rinsed off.

Elasticity: The ability of the skin, tissue, or muscle to return to its original shape.

Elastin: A protein found in the body's dermis and other connective tissue that allows skin to stretch and keep its shape.

Emollient: A softening agent, which helps restore dry skin to a more normal balance.

Estrogen: The hormone responsible for giving women their feminine characteristics. Made predominantly in the ovaries, it has many receptor sites in the female body, including the uterus, vagina, breasts, bones, skin, and even the brain. Estrogen levels vary at different stages of female development, dropping off gradually during perimenopause and declining significantly at menopause.

Extract: The essence of a plant material, drawn out and put in a concentrated form.

Free Radicals: Unstable molecules that attack and destroy cell membranes, speeding aging. Antioxidants can help beat the damage they cause.

Glycerin: A humectant that pulls water from the air and holds it on the skin.

Humectant: An ingredient that holds moisture in the skin or in the hair.

Hypoallergenic: These products are less likely to cause allergic reactions in people than are other similar products in the category. Products classified as hypoallergenic have been shown to have fewer than five people per thousand react to the product.

Kaolin: A naturally occurring clay that absorbs excess oil and is used in skin-care products and masks.

Keratin: A protein found in the skin, hair, teeth, and nails.

Lanolin: The purified fat extracted from the wool of sheep, lanolin makes a great skin conditioner, but can irritate some people's skin.

Liposome: A delivery system formed when certain substances called phospholipids are hydrated in water. The liposomes can absorb and carry various other ingredients and easily penetrate the skin. When the liposomes break down, the ingredients, such as moisturizers, are released into the skin.

Melanin: The natural coloring agents of the skin (that protect it from sun damage). When UV light strikes skin, the skin reacts by producing melanin, or a darker skin tone, commonly known as a tan.

Menopause: The permanent ending of menstruation. The hallmark sign of menopause is the absence of a period for one year.

Mineral Oil: A clear liquid that comes from petroleum and is used for many water-in-oil emulsion moisturizers.

Moisturizer: A product or ingredient that helps build the moisture level of the skin, either by forming a barrier, by stopping the drying out process, or by adding moisture to the skin's layers.

Occlusive: Oils and waxes, such as petrolatum, which form a barrier that water can't penetrate.

Panthenol: A humectant popular for strengthening hair and holding moisture.

pH: The acid or alkaline level of a product. This is determined by how much hydrogen ion is in the ingredients: 7.0 is neutral. Above pH 7.0 is alkaline; below is acidic. Skin normally is acidic, as are hair conditioners. Shampoos and soaps are usually alkaline.

PABA: This sunscreen ingredient absorbs UVB rays, but can cause allergic reactions in some individuals.

Perimenopause: The transitional period that women experience prior to menopause, beginning as early as age 35 and lasting anywhere from four to 15 years (depending on when it begins), until actual menopause occurs.

Photoaging: Reactions to life-time exposure of ultraviolet radiation, which include wrinkles, age spots, loss of skin elasticity, sallow complexion, and broken blood vessels.

Propylene Glycol: A humectant that binds and holds water in the skin; the most common moisture-carrying vehicle in cosmetics, other than water.

Retin-A: The brand name for the cream or gel made from a derivative of vitamin A called tretinoin. Retin-A is available by prescription to treat wrinkles, acne, and sun-damaged skin. It works by making the skin turn over quicker, thus accelerating exfoliation, but it can irritate sensitive skin. It also normalizes skin cell differentiation and maturation, restoring a more youthful appearance. It can also stimulate new collagen, and help to diminish wrinkles.

Sebaceous Glands: The glands in the epidermis that produce sebum, or the skin's natural oils, which trap moisture in the epidermis.

Soap: A product made from animal or vegetable fat that is solid and has an alkaline material added. Soap combines with fatty acids in the skin to remove dirt and grime, but because it strips away the protective oils, it can leave sensitive skin feeling too dry and too tight.

Sodium Lauryl Sulfate: A man-made detergent used in soaps and shampoos that has a very good foaming action.

Squalene: A natural component of human sebum.

Surfactant: These compounds break up oil, grease, and water into small particles so they cleanse better. They can be synthetic or natural, such as from coconut oil. Some are very harsh to the skin.

Tea Tree Oil: A natural substance with antibacterial and anti-inflammatory properties.

Zyderm: An injectable form of bovine collagen.

Zyplast: Same as above. An injectable form of bovine collagen.

Web Sites Worth Looking into

The danger from computers is not that they will eventually get as smart as men, but we will meanwhile agree to meet them halfway.

—BERNARD AVISHAI

The great thing about Web sites is that you can get your hands on a great deal of information in a matter of seconds. Unfortunately, that "immediacy" of information can also pose huge problems, when the information is not quite as credible as you may want it to be (or think it is). How do you separate the wheat from the chaff, then, especially when it comes to something as crucial as your health? Not to worry. To find the most reputable health, skin-care, plastic surgery, medical, and nutrition sites online, I asked Aliza Sherman, Internet Entrepreneur and author of the book *Cybergrrl: A Woman's Guide to the World Wide Web* (Ballantine), http://books.cybergrrl.com, for her help. These are the most credible and reputable Web sites on the topics you most want to look into, plus tantalizing facts and information on the special features of each site. I think you'll also be happy to know that all of the sites listed here are from professional organizations or places of academic study, so it's unlikely you'll run into people trying to sell you products you don't want and definitely don't need.

The Center for Dermatology, Cosmetic and Laser Surgery
http://www.thecenterforderm.com

Dermatology

American Academy for Dermatology
http://www.aad.org/
800-462-DERM (3376)
The site includes professional advice and readily available information on acne. The site can assist you in finding a dermatologist in your area as well as provide you with the latest dermatology news. It even helps you locate a skin cancer screening facility near you for a free cancer screening.

American Society of Dermatology
http://www.asd.org/
309-676-4074
The American Society of Dermatology is dedicated to the preservation of the practice of dermatology, freedom in medicine, and economic freedom. The site includes a membership forum, links, government issues, and current activities. You can even order a T-shirt declaring your support for banning managed care!

American Society of Dermatologic Surgery
http://www.asds-net.org
Professional advice on dermatologic surgery and cosmetic procedures, plus referrals to M.D.s

Dermapathology Inflammatory Diseases of the Skin via Cornell University Medical College
http://edcenter.med.cornell.edu/CUMC_PathNotes/Dermpath/Dermpath_04.html

This is an instructive page of descriptions with links to actual photographs of skin conditions, such as hives, allergic contact dermatitis, and psoriasis. Although the site was last modified on January 11, 1996, the information is still current and correct.

Derm-Infonet
http://www.derm-infonet.com/acnenet/

This site is your friendly source for information on managing a wide variety of skin, hair, and nail disorders. It also provides commonly asked questions and answers about acne. The site links to AcneNet, MelanomaNet, and the American Academy for Dermatology as well as to a teensite, FaceFacts.com, which is sponsored by Roche, the manufacturer of Accutane (a drug used to control acne). You can also use the site to find a dermatologist in your area.

Melanoma Patients Information Page
http://www.sonic.net/~jpat/getwell/or www.mpi.org
800-MRF-1290 (for the Melanoma Research Foundation, which partially funds this Web site)

Contains selected readings tailored to a patient's stage, recommended readings by melanoma patients and their caregivers, an online community and chat room, information about clinical trials, therapy, services, and an archive of articles and abstracts.

National Vitiligo Foundation, Inc.
http://www.nvfi.org/
903-531-0074

NVFI site is a clearinghouse for information about vitiligo, both for people with vitiligo and for the general public. It contains several resources, including a list of physicians, support services, a treatment library, and a vitiligo study. The site includes a link to buy a book titled *Different Just Like Me*, written by a mother of a child with vitiligo. The book covers all the ways that people are different (short, tall, handicapped, old, young) from a child's viewpoint.

Psoriasis.org
http://www.psoriasis.org/
503-244-7404

Provides information about psoriasis, including articles on research, therapies, and the latest news as well as National Psoriasis Foundation (NPF) services, publications, and events. One section, Just4Us, deals with the issues and questions facing kids and teens with psoriasis, plus fun stuff like free posters to download, poetry and short stories sent in by kids and teens, and articles to read. Another section on the site lists volunteer activities, and there is even a place for families to respond who want to get involved in psoriasis research.

Rosacea.org
http://www.rosacea.org/
1-888-NO-BLUSH

This site provides a complete description on what rosacea is and how to treat it as well as information about their hotline and other services. The site also gives a listing of links to other related Web sites, offers issues of *Rosacea Review*, a newsletter for rosacea sufferers, and provides a list of "trigger" factors that can influence rosacea, including food, weather conditions, and medical conditions. The site also includes a history of rosacea, including its first diagnosis by a fourteenth-century French physician, who called it "goutterose" (French for "pink droplet"), and early treatments, which included bloodletting and applying leeches.

Skin Savvy
http://www.aad.org/ss98/ss98index.html

This fun site, brought to you by the American Academy of Dermatology, is chock full of information. It includes a quiz to determine your skin cancer risk and information about Camp Discovery, a week-long summer camp for children with severe skin conditions. The site also offers a useful list of articles provided by the American Academy of Dermatology that includes statistics, a primer on adult acne, and a guide to skin self-exams.

General Health

Discovery Health
http://www.discoveryhealth.com/

This informative site offers the latest on health issues. It includes an extensive question-and-answer section, many health topics (including alternative health and seniors' health), and text of articles in scientific publications. An added bonus: great forums, related sites, a good search engine, reference rooms, and personnel advice given by the experts. You can also access videos that go with articles.

Dr. Koop
http://www.drkoop.com/

This site showcases the information of Dr. C. Everett Koop, former U.S. Surgeon General, as well as others who are dedicated to improving the quality of people's lives by empowering them to improve their health. The site covers a wide range of health topics, including top news stories, prevention, support groups, and live chats. It also includes calculators (interactive tools to help you get better health), insurance information, a good search engine, and recalls of consumer products.

Medical

Doctor Finder via the AMA (American Medical Association)
http://www.ama-assn.org/aps/amahg.htm
312-464-5000 (AMA headquarters)

This is an easy-to-use searchable database, where you can search for a doctor by name or medical specialty—for example, for pediatricians specifically—or you can search through their Reference Library for health information on specific conditions.

Mediconsult
http://www.mediconsult.com/

This fun, easy-to-use site contains comprehensive "condition centers" with reliable, in-depth information. Their mission is to provide timely, comprehensive, and accessible medical information on chronic medical conditions. They are independent of any hospital, drug company, HMO, hospital, or other health-care organization to ensure unbiased, objective, and credible information. All information on their site goes through a rigorous clinical review process.

Medscape
http://www.medscape.com/

This site provides daily health news, which includes great medical information for patients, students, and doctors. Site destinations include specialty home pages for various medical issues (such as diabetes, cardiology, oncology, primary care), and it also covers conferences on a variety of health topics.

National Health Information Center
http://nhic-nt.health.org/

NHIC is a health information referral service, and the site contains a Health Information Resource Database (with 2,000 toll-free numbers for health information), announcements, publications, and links to 1,100 organizations and government offices that provide health information upon request.

National Institutes of Health Search Engine (NIH)
http://search.info.nih.gov

This is a powerful search engine into a vast medical and health database. It includes articles from the National Library of Medicine's MedLine Plus and other government health resources as well as general information on topics ranging from tanning to dry skin.

Nutrition

American Dietetic Association
http://www.eatright.org/
800-366-1655

This is a fun Web site, offering a lot of sound nutrition information, hot topics, child nutrition and health, food guide pyramids (children's, as well), quizzes, book excerpts, and advice on how to find a registered dietitian in your area.

American Heart Association
Visit the main site at http://www.americanheart.org/ or check out http://www.deliciousdecisions.org/
800-AHA-USA1 (Customer Heart and Stroke Information)
1-888-MY-HEART (Women's Health Information)
The American Heart Association provides visitors with tips for improved eating and living habits as well as access to a database of recipes that are low in fat, cholesterol, and sodium to promote good nutrition. It also provides links to other Web sites and pages.

Plastic Surgery

American Academy of Facial Plastic and Reconstructive Surgery
http://www.facial-plastic-surgery.org
703-299-9291
AAFPRS is the world's largest organization of facial plastic and reconstructive surgeons and the only organization dedicated to the advancement of the highest quality of facial plastic and reconstructive surgery. The site includes helpful areas like Patient Information, Facial Plastic Surgery Today (a consumer newsletter), and a Member Directory.

American Board of Plastic and Reconstructive Surgery
http://www.abfprs.org
703-549-3223
Established in 1986, ABFPRS is dedicated to improving the quality of facial plastic surgery available to the public by measuring the qualifications of candidate surgeons against certain rigorous standards.

The American Society for Plastic Surgeons (formerly the American Society for Plastic and Reconstructive Surgeons),
www.plasticsurgery.org.
847-228-9900

This is the group associated with the American Board of Plastic Surgeons, who are responsible for the board-certification of plastic surgeons. You can find a plastic surgeon, see a video about insurance coverage of plastic repair of children's congentital defects, and learn about the evolution of plastic surgery.

Foundation for Reconstructive Plastic Surgery
http://www.frps.org
212-794-1234
A nonprofit organization whose mission is the promotion of excellence in plastic surgery through professional and public education, FRPS provides information on finding a surgeon (including ways to see whether you are eligible for "pro bono" surgery) and educational software. FRPS also has a speaker's bureau from which you can request a plastic surgeon to speak to your organization or club meeting.

Services

The American Cancer Society
http://www.cancer.org
800-ACS-2345
The American Cancer Society can provide you with skin-care information and support. The hardworking site includes a patient service section, the latest fundraising news, a wide variety of related links, suggested books to read, and information on alternative methods of treatment.

Botanical Dermatology Database
http://BoDD.cf.ac.uk/Indexes/PlantFamilies.html
Based on the book *Botanical Dermatology*, by J. Mitchell and A. Rook, which was originally published in 1979 by Greengrass Ltd, Vancouver [ISBN 0-88978-047-1], this site contains detailed scientific information about plants. It also offers an extensive alphabetical list of plant families, including details about the plants, what substances are derived from them, and how they might affect your skin.

Environmental Protection Agency
http://www.epa.gov/
202-260-2090

The EPA's mission is to protect human health and to safeguard the natural environment. The EPA site includes informational resources for kids, students, teachers, concerned citizens, researchers, scientists, small business, and industry. Information includes projects, programs, news, laws and regulations, offices and labs, and publications.

FDA Center for Food Safety and Nutrition
http://vm.cfsan.fda.gov/list.html

The FDA provides a variety of food safety and nutrition information. The site includes an overview of the FDA's history, different program areas, sections on cosmetics, dietary supplements, the latest press releases, and offers a way to get in touch with the FDA to report complaints with foods or cosmetics products.

Cosmetic Products (via the FDA)
http://vm.cfsan.fda.gov/~dms/cos-cfr.html

This site provides general enforcement regulations, administrative rulings and decisions, and other public information from the FDA regarding cosmetics products.

Mayo Health Oasis
http://www.mayohealth.org/

This excellent, easy-to-use site, which is updated daily and produced by the Mayo Clinic, includes sections on allergies, cancer, nutrition, and other health-related articles, as well as news of medical breakthroughs and discoveries. The Mayo Clinic's Women's Health Center offers health quizzes to test your knowledge, articles covering women's health issues, and the opportunity to get answers to your most pressing health questions from doctors of the Mayo Clinic.

Skin Cancer (at the Mayo Clinic)
http://www.mayo.ivi.com/mayo/9403/htm/skincanc.htm

Provides very basic information about skin cancer from a trusted source.

National Institutes of Health
http://www.nih.gov/

This biomedical research center offers health information, a wide range of consumer health publications, and a subject word guide to diseases and conditions that the NIH is investigating.

The Center for Dermatology, Cosmetic and Laser Surgery
http://www.thecenterforderm.com
914-241-3003

This is the web site for my practice, located in Mount Kisco, NY. I and my colleagues (three other dermatologists and a plastic surgeon, all board certified) offer a one-stop resource for all dermatological concerns and cosmetic procedures. You can find out more about the doctors' training and background, see more before and after photos of the procedures we do, buy skin care products online, and find out what's new and exciting for skin care and appearance enhancement.

Index